OXFORD HIGHER SPECIALTY TRAINING

OSCEs for Intensive Care Medicine

OXFORD HIGHER SPECIALTY TRAINING

OSCEs for Intensive Care Medicine

Dr Peter Hersey MBChB MMEd CertMgmt EDIC FRCA FFICM
Consultant in Intensive Care Medicine and Anaesthesia
South Tyneside and Sunderland NHS Foundation Trust
Sunderland, UK

Dr Laura O'Connor MBChB MRCP FRCA FFICM
Consultant in Intensive Care Medicine and Anaesthesia
South Tyneside and Sunderland NHS Foundation Trust
Sunderland, UK

Dr Tom Sams MBChB MRCP FRCA FFICM
Consultant in Intensive Care Medicine and Anaesthesia
North Cumbria Integrated Care NHS Foundation Trust
Carlisle, UK

Dr Jon Sturman MBChB MRCP EDIC FRCA DCh FFICM
Consultant in Intensive Care Medicine and Anaesthesia
North Cumbria Integrated Care NHS Foundation Trust
Carlisle, UK

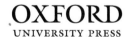

OXFORD
UNIVERSITY PRESS

UNIVERSITY PRESS

Great Clarendon Street, Oxford, OX2 6DP,
United Kingdom

Oxford University Press is a department of the University of Oxford.
It furthers the University's objective of excellence in research, scholarship,
and education by publishing worldwide. Oxford is a registered trade mark of
Oxford University Press in the UK and in certain other countries

© Oxford University Press 2020

The moral rights of the authors have been asserted

First Edition published in 2020

Impression: 1

Published in the United States of America by Oxford University Press
198 Madison Avenue, New York, NY 10016, United States of America

British Library Cataloguing in Publication Data

Data available

Library of Congress Control Number: 2020938137

ISBN 978–0–19–882437–4

Printed and bound by
CPI Group (UK) Ltd, Croydon, CR0 4YY

PH: For George and Seth

LOC: For Anne and Vincent

TS: For Charlie and Zoe

About the Authors

Dr Peter Hersey MBChB MMEd CertMgmt EDIC FRCA FFICM

Peter is the clinical lead for critical care at South Tyneside and Sunderland NHSFT and a previous FICM Faculty Tutor. He undertakes both local and national roles in medical education. After taking up his consultant post he was awarded a postgraduate masters in medical education, and was the founding director for a course preparing candidates for the final FFICM OSCE.

Dr Laura O'Connor MBChB MRCP FRCA FFICM

Laura is a consultant and FICM Faculty Tutor in Sunderland Royal Hospital where she also leads an active simulation programme. She has experience of working in New Zealand and holds the FFICM by examination.

Dr Tom Sams MBChB MRCP FRCA FFICM

Tom trained in Sheffield and Newcastle before taking up his consultant post at North Cumbria NHSFT. He is a FICM Faculty Tutor and has organized several successful revision courses. He was one of the first candidates to sit the final FFICM examination.

Dr Jon Sturman MBChB MRCP EDIC FRCA DCh FFICM

Jon takes an active role in multiprofessional training both within the UK and abroad and has an interest in developing remote and rural intensive care. After training which included a fellowship in paediatric retrieval, he took a consultant post at North Cumbria NHSFT, where he has been clinical director since 2012.

Contents

Abbreviations

ABG	arterial blood gas
ACS	abdominal compartment syndrome
AECOPD	acute exacerbations of chronic obstructive pulmonary disease
AF	atrial fibrillation
AFLD	acute fatty liver disease
ALP	alkaline phosphatase
ALT	alanine aminotransferase
AOF	atrio-oesophageal fistula
ARR	absolute risk reduction
AST	aspartate aminotransferase
AV	atrioventricular
BE	base excess
BNP	brain natriuretic peptide
BP	blood pressure
bpm	beats per minute
CDI	*Clostridium difficile* infection
CIM	critical illness myopathy
CIP	critical illness polyneuropathy
CN	cranial nerve
CoBaTrICE	Competency-Based Training in Intensive Care Medicine in Europe
COPD	chronic obstructive pulmonary disease
CPR	cardiopulmonary resuscitation
CSF	cerebrospinal fluid
CT	computed tomography
CTIMP	clinical trial of an investigational medicinal product
CTPA	computed tomography pulmonary angiogram
CVP	central venous pressure
DAS	Difficult Airway Society
DC	direct current
DH	decompressive hemicraniectomy
DLCO	lung diffusion capacity for carbon monoxide
DOAC	direct oral anticoagulant
ECMO	extracorporeal membrane oxygenation
EDIC	European Diploma in Intensive Care Medicine
EEG	electroencephalogram
ERCP	endoscopic retrograde cholangiopancreatogram
ETT	endotracheal tube
FEV_1	forced expiratory volume in 1 second
FFICM	Fellowship of the Faculty of Intensive Care Medicine
FiO_2	fraction of inspired oxygen
FVC	forced vital capacity
GGT	gamma-glutamyl transferase
Hb	haemoglobin
HCO_3^-	bicarbonate
HELLP	haemolysis, elevated liver enzymes, and low platelets
HFNO	high-flow nasal oxygen

HIT	heparin-induced thrombocytopenia
HIV	human immunodeficiency virus
HRCT	high-resolution computed tomography
IABP	intra-aortic balloon pump
IAH	intra-abdominal hypertension
IAP	intra-abdominal pressure
ICD	implantable cardioverter defibrillator
ICP	measure intracranial pressure
ICUAW	intensive care unit-associated weakness
IE	infective endocarditis
Ig	immunoglobulin
IM	intramuscular
INR	international normalized ratio
IO	intraosseous
IV	intravenous
LDH	lactate dehydrogenase
LMWH	low-molecular-weight heparin
LT	double-lumen tube
LVAD	left ventricular assist device
MCA	middle cerebral artery
MCV	mean cell volume
MPH	massive pulmonary haemorrhage
MRCP	magnetic resonance cholangiopancreatography
MRI	magnetic resonance imaging
MT	Minnesota tube
NAC	N-acetylcysteine
NEX	nose–ear–xiphisternum
NG	nasogastric
NHS	National Health Service
NHSI	NHS Improvement
NICE	National Institute for Health and Care Excellence
NIV	non-invasive ventilation
NNT	number needed to treat
NT	N terminal
OI	oxygenation index
OSCE	objective structured clinical examination
PA	pulmonary artery
PAC	pulmonary artery catheter
PAH	pulmonary arterial hypertension
PaO_2	partial pressure of oxygen
PAOP	pulmonary artery occlusion pressure
PCI	primary percutaneous intervention
PCO_2	partial pressure of carbon dioxide
PE	pulmonary embolism
PEEP	positive end-expiratory pressure
PF4	platelet factor 4
qSOFA	quick sequential organ failure assessment score
RRR	relative risk reduction
RSBI	rapid shallow breathing index
RSV	respiratory syncytial virus
RV	right ventricle/ventricular

RVAD	right ventricular assist device
SAD	supraglottic airway device
SBE	standard base excess
SBP	systolic blood pressure
SBT	Sengstaken–Blakemore tube or spontaneous breathing trial
$ScvO_2$	central venous oxygen saturation
SpO_2	peripheral capillary oxygen saturation
STEMI	ST elevation myocardial infarction
SVC	superior vena cava
SvO_2	mixed venous saturation
TB	tuberculosis
TBSA	total body surface area
TCA	tricyclic antidepressant
TLC	total lung capacity
TLS	tumour lysis syndrome
TPN	total parenteral nutrition
VA	venoarterial
VAD	ventricular assist device
VF	ventricular fibrillation
VHA	viscoelastic haemostatic assay
VT	ventricular tachycardia
VV	venovenous
WCC	white cell count

Introduction

Passing the Fellowship of the Faculty of Intensive Care Medicine (FFICM) examination is a requirement of the UK training programme in intensive care medicine. Similarly, to be awarded the European Diploma in Intensive Care Medicine (EDIC) a doctor must demonstrate the specialist knowledge required for the intensive care clinician. Objective structured clinical examination (OSCE) components can prove to be a problematic hurdle even for doctors with several years of clinical experience and who are experienced in sitting postgraduate exams.

We think that difficulties in practising for this style of examination can be a reason for poor performance on the day itself. This book has been written to help candidates prepare for the OSCE by providing a bank of practice questions organized into practice exams. We have mapped the questions not only to the UK syllabus for training in intensive care medicine but also to the European equivalent: Competency-Based Training in Intensive Care Medicine in Europe (CoBaTrICE).

The questions have been written to cover as much of the syllabus as possible but also to highlight some areas that appear more frequently in exams than in day-to-day practice. We have used our experiences of sitting and observing the final FFICM exam and of running a successful FFICM OSCE preparation course to produce a resource that will give candidates the confidence to perform at their very best when it really matters.

While the book will be most useful for those about to sit the exam, the questions will also be useful as a resource for those planning bedside teaching or simply wanting to improve their knowledge of intensive care medicine. This includes candidates preparing for the second part examination towards Fellowship of the College of Intensive Care Medicine of Australia and New Zealand.

How to Use This Book

- This book contains 104 questions, divided into eight OSCEs. As with the FFICM final OSCE, they cover the themes of professionalism, resuscitation, data interpretation, and equipment. The proportion of questions for each theme is the same as in the exam.
- As with the exam itself, the questions have been written to avoid 'double jeopardy'. Avoiding double jeopardy means that if you don't know the answer to part of a question you can still achieve all subsequent marks. Because of this, it's vitally important that you don't read ahead when answering questions. Double jeopardy is also the reason why examiners won't go back to an earlier question once it's 'asked and answered'.
- While some of the questions in the book will be straightforward, some will appear difficult. Remember that you would not be expected to achieve all 20 marks to pass an OSCE station (the pass mark will depend on the difficulty of the question). The questions have been written so that the reader will increase their knowledge as well as revising what is already known.
- The book is written to be a useful resource to help you to pass the exam—please don't get stressed about anything within it. Postgraduate exams are not fun, but rest assured they will soon be over, and this will all become a distant memory.

Our Tips for Success

- The syllabus describes what you can be asked, so read it early to plan your learning. Try to avoid just learning what you find interesting or easy, and remember that having a broad knowledge with few gaps will serve you better than having detailed knowledge in fewer areas.
- After each sitting of the FFICM OSCE, the chief examiner produces a report. Included within it are descriptions of when and how candidates performed poorly. Being familiar with it is the best way of learning from other people's experiences.
- Try and gain as much varied clinical exposure as possible. Candidates can struggle with subspecialty questions if they've not had this experience.
- The OSCE is meant to replicate the world of work. Talking through your day-to-day activities with colleagues is an excellent OSCE practice. What could you be asked about the task you've just completed? How would you explain what you've just done?
- Remember the basics for the easy marks.
- If you don't know, you don't know. While it is often worth an educated guess, you should concentrate on the marks that are still available.
- You will undoubtedly be faced with electrocardiograms and imaging, so it's well worth practising a systematic approach you can rely on.
- Once you've completed a station, forget about it. No matter how (you think) you've performed, it's in the past and you have the next station to concentrate on.
- Dress smartly but comfortably. If a station needs you to do something (e.g. resuscitation, examination), don't be afraid to take off your jacket.
- The OSCE can be noisy. Try to ignore the candidate shouting out answers in the next booth or any movement going on outside.
- Remember that the examiners want you to pass.
- Listen to the question and do what's asked. If you don't understand the question, ask for it to be repeated.
- And the hardest thing of all … stay calm!

Good luck!

OSCE 1

OSCE 1 station 1—professionalism

Questions

You are asked to speak to the family of a patient (John) who has been admitted to the intensive care unit with a severe brain injury. Overnight, a repeat computed tomography scan of the head showed expansion of the intracranial haemorrhage. On the ward round, John was noted to have bilateral dilated pupils, absent spontaneous respiratory effort, and no cough reflex. The family are aware that a deterioration has occurred.

You plan to carry out brainstem death testing and go to speak to John's wife. She asks the following questions:

a) 'Can you explain what has happened?' *(4 marks)*
b) 'What do the tests involve?' *(6 marks)*
c) 'What do you think the tests will show?' *(1 mark)*
d) 'How can someone be dead when their heart is still beating and he is warm?' *(4 marks)*

Answers

a) 'Can you explain what has happened?' *(4 marks)*
  - Clarify the relatives' existing knowledge and understanding of the current situation
  - Explain that further bleeding has occurred which you think has resulted in further brain damage
  - Explain that you suspect that the patient has lost the ability to ever regain consciousness or breathe for themselves. You plan tests to confirm that this is the case
  - State that if the patient has lost the ability to ever regain consciousness or breathe for themselves, they have died

b) 'What do the tests involve?' *(6 marks)*
  - Brainstem death tests are a clinical examination conducted at the bedside by two senior doctors
  - The examination is only carried out when certain conditions have been met. This is to avoid misleading results
  - The examination is conducted twice
  - As part of the examination, John will be disconnected from the ventilator to see if he can breathe
  - The family can be present to observe the tests
  - Reflex movements can sometimes occur; these can be unexpected but will be explained

c) 'What do you think the tests will show?' *(1 mark)*
  - You expect that the tests will show that John has died

d) 'How can John be dead when his heart is still beating and he is warm?' *(4 marks)*
  - Death occurs when the brain has lost its essential functions, which are the ability to breathe and to regain consciousness
  - John is not conscious, and his breathing is being performed entirely by the ventilator
  - His heart doesn't need his brain to be functioning to beat; it just needs oxygen which the ventilator is providing. If we disconnected the ventilator, oxygen levels would fall and his heart would stop beating
  - John feels warm because his heart is still pumping warm blood around his body

General communication *(5 marks)*

Marks awarded for behaviours such as the following:
  - Eye contact, introduces self, and body language
  - Pace and volume of speech
  - Demonstrates empathy and addresses concerns
  - Offers clear explanations
  - Avoids medical jargon

Notes

It may be tempting to showcase your medical knowledge to the examiner by providing an in-depth account of the performance of brainstem death testing. However, remember that this is a communication skills station and it is your interaction with the actor as well as your knowledge that is being examined. If the actor asks you a question it will be for a reason.

The words and phrases you use will differ from what is written here, but the mark scheme represents the key messages that you would be expected to give.

Further reading

Academy of Medical Royal Colleges. A code of practice for the diagnosis and confirmation of death. 2008. Available at: http://www.aomrc.org.uk/wp-content/uploads/2016/04/Code_Practice_Confirmation_Diagnosis_Death_1008-4.pdf [accessed 4 December 2017].

FFICM syllabus references 3.6, 7.1, 8.1, 8.2, 8.4, 12.1, 12.4, 12.12.
CoBaTrICE domains 2, 8, 12.

OSCE 1 station 2—resuscitation

Questions

You are called to see a patient on the ward who has a return of spontaneous circulation following a cardiac arrest. The patient is groaning.

a) How would you assess the patient? *(4 marks)*

On initial assessment you find:

- Patent airway
- Bilateral equal chest movement with good air entry, respiratory rate 18 breaths/minute, SpO_2 94% on high-flow oxygen
- Heart rate 45 beats per minute (regular), poor pulse volume, blood pressure 57/30 mmHg
- Alert to voice, capillary glucose 5.5 (3.5–5.5 mmol/L)

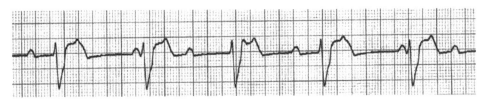

Figure 1.1 Rhythm strip

Reproduced from *Oxford Handbook of Cardiac Nursing, Second Edition*, Olson K, et al., Figure 11.6. © 2014 Oxford University Press. Reproduced with permission of the Licensor through PLSclear

You are handed the rhythm strip from the defibrillator. Look at Figure 1.1.

b) What is the rhythm, and what syndrome is the patient suffering from? *(2 marks)*
c) Complete the missing text in Figure 1.2 to describe the management of bradycardia *(12 marks)*
d) Other than transvenous pacing, what other pacing techniques can be used? *(2 marks)*

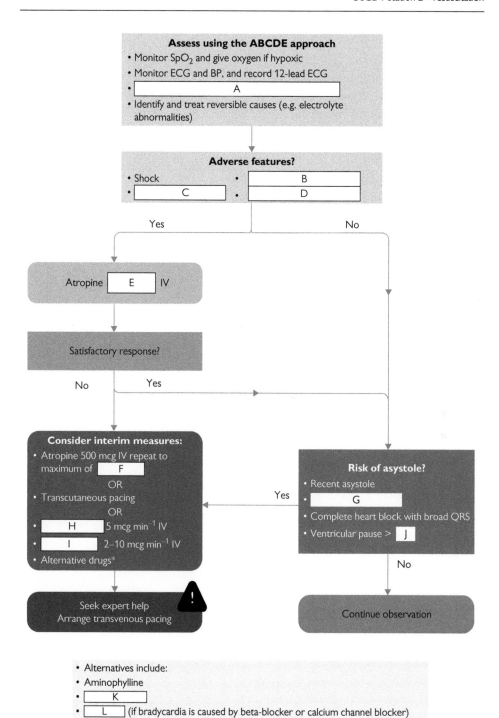

Figure 1.2 Bradycardia treatment algorithm

Reproduced with the kind permission of the Resuscitation Council (UK)

Answers

a) How would you assess the patient? *(4 marks)*
   - Assess airway patency—look, listen, and feel
   - Assess breathing—chest movement and deformity, air entry, SpO_2, respiratory rate, cyanosis
   - Assess circulation—capillary refill time, blood pressure, colour, peripheral and central pulses (rate and rhythm)
   - Assess disability—Glasgow Coma Score or AVPU ('alert, verbal, pain, unresponsive'), capillary glucose

b) What is the rhythm, and what syndrome is the patient suffering from? *(2 marks)*
   - Complete heart block
   - Cardiogenic shock

c) Complete the missing text in Figure 1.2 to describe the management of bradycardia *(12 marks)*
   - A. Obtain intravenous access
   - B. Myocardial ischaemia
   - C. Syncope
   - D. Heart failure
   - E. 500 mcg
   - F. 3 mg
   - G. Mobitz II atrioventricular block
   - H. Isoprenaline
   - I. Adrenaline
   - J. 3 seconds
   - K. Dopamine
   - L. Glucagon

d) Other than transvenous pacing, what other pacing techniques can be used? *(2 marks)*
   - Transcutaneous pacing
   - Fist (percussion) pacing

Further reading

Resuscitation Council (UK). Resuscitation guidelines. Available at: https://www.resus.org.uk/resuscitation-guidelines [accessed 15 October 2018].

FFICM syllabus references, 1.1, 1.2, 1.3, 2.1, 2.3, 2.7, 3.1, 3.3, 4.1, 4.4, 4.5, 5.1, 5.12, 12.2, 12.7, 12.9, 12.11. **CoBaTrICE domains** 1, 2, 3, 4, 5.

OSCE 1 station 3—data

Questions

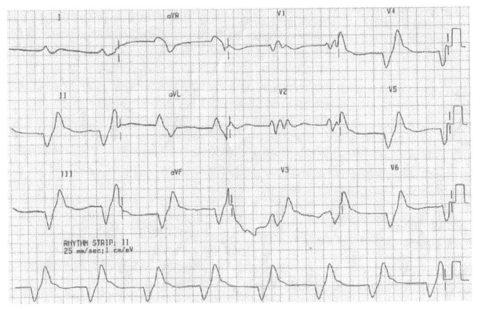

Figure 1.3 Electrocardiogram (ECG)

Reproduced from *Oxford Textbook of Medicine, Fifth Edition*, Warrell D, et al. (eds). Firth J, Acute Kidney Injury, Figure 21.5.3. © 2010 Oxford University Press. Reproduced with permission of the Licensor through PLSclear

Look at Figure 1.3.

a) Describe this ECG *(5 marks)*
b) What is the most likely cause for this ECG appearance? *(1 mark)*
c) How is severe hyperkalaemia defined? *(1 mark)*
d) What cardiac rhythm would the patient be most likely to progress to if hyperkalaemia is left untreated? *(1 mark)*
e) Complete Table 1.1q regarding the mechanism of action of drugs causing hyperkalaemia *(4 marks)*

Table 1.1q Mechanisms of drug-induced hyperkalaemia

Mechanism of action	Example medication
Impaired potassium distribution	
Increased total body potassium	
Reduced renal potassium excretion	
Affects the renin–angiotensin system	

f) What is pseudohyperkalaemia? *(1 mark)*
g) What are the possible causes of pseudohyperkalaemia? *(3 marks)*

h) Complete Table 1.2q regarding the mechanisms of action of treatments for hyperkalaemia *(4 marks)*

Table 1.2q Mechanisms of action of hyperkalaemia treatments

Mechanism of action	Treatment
	Calcium chloride, calcium gluconate
	Insulin, sodium bicarbonate, beta agonists, e.g. salbutamol
	Furosemide, haemodialysis/haemofiltration
	Cation exchange resins, e.g. sodium or calcium polystyrene sulphonate

Answers

a) Describe this ECG *(5 marks)*
  - Regular
  - Bradycardia, 42 beats per minute
  - Large, tented T waves
  - Absent P waves
  - Widened QRS
b) What is the most likely cause for this ECG appearance? *(1 mark)*
  - Severe hyperkalaemia
c) How is severe hyperkalaemia defined? *(1 mark)*
  - A serum potassium concentration above 7.0 mmol/L or
  - A patient with symptoms or ECG changes
d) What cardiac rhythm would the patient be most likely to progress to if hyperkalaemia is left untreated? *(1 mark)*
  - Ventricular fibrillation
e) Complete Table 1.1a regarding the mechanism of action of drugs causing hyperkalaemia *(4 marks)*

Table 1.1a Mechanisms of drug-induced hyperkalaemia

Mechanism of action	Example medication
Impaired potassium distribution	Digoxin, beta blockers, suxamethonium, arginine
Increased total body potassium	Potassium supplements (Sando K®), intravenous fluids containing potassium
Reduced renal potassium excretion	Calcineurin inhibitors (tacrolimus and ciclosporin), potassium-sparing diuretics, trimethoprim
Affects the renin–angiotensin system	Non-steroidal anti-inflammatory drugs (NSAIDs), angiotensin-converting enzyme (ACE) inhibitors, angiotensin-II receptor inhibitors, heparin

f) What is pseudohyperkalaemia? *(1 mark)*
  - A phenomenon whereby the measured serum potassium concentration is higher than the true value
g) What are the possible causes of pseudohyperkalaemia? *(3 marks)*

  (1 mark per cause to a maximum of 3)
  - Test tube haemolysis
  - Tight tourniquet with or without exercise
  - Leukaemia with high white cell count
  - Thrombocytosis

h) Complete Table 1.2a regarding the mechanisms of action of treatments for hyperkalaemia
   (4 marks)

Table 1.2a Mechanisms of action of hyperkalaemia treatments

Mechanism of action	Treatment
Membrane stabilization	Calcium chloride, calcium gluconate
Intracellular shift of potassium	Insulin, sodium bicarbonate, beta agonists, e.g. salbutamol
Increased elimination	Furosemide, haemodialysis/haemofiltration
Binding in the gastrointestinal tract	Cation exchange resins, e.g. sodium or calcium polystyrene sulphonate

Further reading

Firth JD. Acute kidney injury. In: Warrell DA, Cox TM, Firth JD (eds.) *Oxford Textbook of Medicine*, 5th Edition, pp. 3385–3903. Oxford: Oxford University Press; 2010.

FFICM syllabus references 1.1, 2.3, 2.8, 3.1, 3.4, 3.10, 4.1, 4.8.
CoBaTrICE domains 2, 3.

OSCE 1 station 4—data

Questions

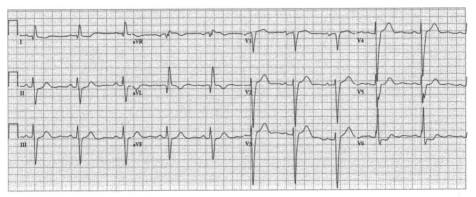

Figure 1.4 Electrocardiogram (ECG)

Reproduced from *The Brigham Intensive Review of Internal Medicine*, Singh AK and Loscalzo J, Figure 86.9. © 2014 Oxford University Press. Reproduced with permission of the Licensor through PLSclear

Look at Figure 1.4.

a) What abnormalities are shown on this ECG? *(6 marks)*

b) What is the normal axis for left ventricular depolarization in an adult? *(1 mark)*

c) What is a 'strain pattern', and why is it important? *(2 marks)*

d) With respect to left ventricular hypertrophy (LVH), what are the Sokolow–Lyon criteria? *(2 marks)*

e) What is the most common cause of LVH? *(1 mark)*

f) How might transthoracic echocardiography be useful in a patient with ECG criteria for LVH? *(5 marks)*

g) What are the potential adverse clinical consequences of non-obstructive LVH? *(3 marks)*

Answers

a) What abnormalities are shown on this ECG? *(6 marks)*
  - Left axis deviation
  - Tall R waves in V6
  - Deep S waves in V2–5
  - Broad QRS complexes
  - Non-specific QRS morphology abnormalities
  - ST segment depression in V6

b) What is the normal axis for left ventricular depolarization in an adult? *(1 mark)*
  - −30 to +90 degrees

c) What is a 'strain pattern', and why is it important? *(2 marks)*
  - ST segment depression and asymmetrical negative T waves in the lateral precordial leads
  - Patients with this pattern have an increased risk of cardiovascular morbidity and mortality

d) With respect to left ventricular hypertrophy (LVH), what are the Sokolow–Lyon criteria? *(2 marks)*

  (1 mark for a correct but incomplete answer)
  - LVH should be suspected if the combined amplitude of the R wave in V5 or V6 plus the S wave in V1 or V2 is >35 mm, or if the R wave in aVL is ≥11 mm

e) What is the most common cause of LVH? *(1 mark)*
  - Hypertension

f) How might transthoracic echocardiography be useful in a patient with ECG criteria for LVH? *(5 marks)*
  - To measure ventricular wall thickness (to confirm the diagnosis and to diagnose idiopathic hypertrophic cardiomyopathy)
  - To assess valvular function
  - To assess systolic and diastolic ventricular function
  - To diagnose aortic coarctation and assess for other causes of outflow obstruction
  - To assess the response to treatment in patients with LVH caused by hypertension

g) What are the potential adverse clinical consequences of non-obstructive LVH? *(3 marks)*
  - Cardiac failure
  - Ischaemic heart disease
  - Arrhythmias

Further reading

Lorell BH, Carabello BA. Left ventricular hypertrophy. *Circulation* 2000;102:470–479.

FFICM syllabus references 2.2, 2.3, 3.2, 3.3.
CoBaTrICE domain 2.

OSCE 1 station 5—data

Questions

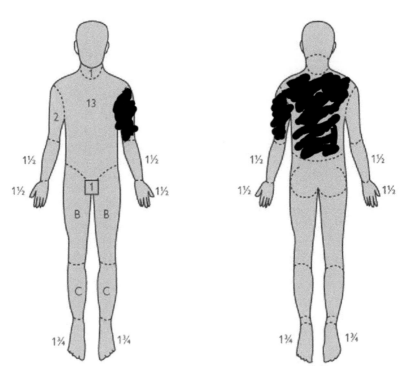

AREA	Age 0	1	5	10	15	Adult
A-1½ OF HEAD	9½	8½	6½	5½	4½	3½
B-1½ OF ONE HEAD	2¾	3¼	4	4½	4½	4¾
C-½ OF ONE LOWER LEG	2½	2½	2¾	3	3¼	3½

Figure 1.5 Emergency department documentation

Lund CC, Browder NC. The estimation of areas of burns. *Surgery Gynecology & Obstetrics* 1944;79:352–358. From the Journal of the American College of Surgeons, formerly *Surgery Gycecology & Obstetrics*. Reprinted with permission from the Journal of the American College of Surgeons, formerly *Surgery Gynecology & Obstetrics*

A healthy adult is brought to the emergency department having fallen onto a bonfire. To document the extent of their burn injury, the chart shown in Figure 1.5 was completed.

a) By what name is the chart in Figure 1.5 commonly known? *(1 mark)*
b) What percentage of total body surface area (TBSA) is affected by the burn? *(1 mark)*
c) What other methods are available to estimate the TBSA affected by a burn? *(2 marks)*

The burn on the patient's arm is noted to be non-blanching. The burn on the patient's back is painful and blisters are beginning to form.

d) What emergency surgical procedure may be required? *(1 mark)*

e) What percentage TBSA burn would meet the criterial for referral to a burns centre on area alone? *(1 mark)*

f) On what criteria should this patient be given intravenous fluid resuscitation? *(1 mark)*

g) Describe the Parkland formula for intravenous fluid replacement after a burn *(3 marks)*

The patient has a carboxyhaemoglobin level of 5%.

h) Would they be considered to have suffered an inhalation injury? *(2 marks)*

i) What features in a patient with burns would indicate a need for early intubation? *(6 marks)*

j) When is it safe to use suxamethonium after a significant burn injury? *(2 marks)*

Answers

a) By what name is the chart in Figure 1.5 commonly known? *(1 mark)*
   - Lund and Browder chart
b) What percentage of total body surface area (TBSA) is affected by the burn? *(1 mark)*
   - 17%
c) What other methods are available to estimate the TBSA affected by a burn? *(2 marks)*
   - Wallace's rule of 9s
   - Palm of the patient's hand = 1% TBSA
d) What emergency surgical procedure may be required? *(1 mark)*
   - Escharotomies of the arm
e) What percentage TBSA burn would meet the criteria for referral to a burns centre on area alone? *(1 mark)*
   - >40%
f) On what criteria should this patient be given intravenous fluid resuscitation? *(1 mark)*
   - Burn >15% TBSA
g) Describe the Parkland formula for intravenous fluid replacement after a burn *(3 marks)*
   - Crystalloid (Ringer's lactate was originally described)
   - 4 mL/kg/%TBSA over 24 hours
   - Half the volume is given in the first 8 hours following the injury
h) Would they be considered to have suffered an inhalation injury? *(2 marks)*
   - No, levels of up to 10% can be seen in smokers and in urban environments
   - Also, the injury was sustained in an open environment
i) What features of a patient with burns would indicate a need for early intubation? *(6 marks)*
   - Voice changes (hoarse voice or stridor)
   - Singed nasal hair or carbonaceous sputum
   - Visible swelling or blistering of the lips, tongue, or oropharynx
   - Deep burns to the face/neck
   - Respiratory distress or failure
   - Glasgow Coma Scale score of <8
j) When is it safe to use suxamethonium after a significant burn injury? *(2 marks)*

   - Within the first 24 hours
   - After 1 year post burn

Notes

These questions in part relate to UK arrangements for burn care, so those sections would not be applicable elsewhere.

Further reading

National Network for Burn Care. National Burn Care referral guidance. 2012. Available at: https://www.britishburnassociation.org/national-burn-care-referral-guidance [accessed 22 January 2018].

FFICM syllabus references 1.6, 2.1, 2.5, 12.7.
CoBaTrICE domains 1, 2, 3.

OSCE 1 station 6—data

Questions

A 74-year-old man was admitted to the intensive care unit following an emergency laparotomy for a perforated large bowel with extensive peritoneal soiling. Postoperatively he has been sedated and ventilated and has required vasopressor support.

On your review you note that over the last 12 hours he has developed:

- Reducing urine output and a 350% increase in creatinine compared to admission
- Increasing vasopressor requirements despite optimal fluid status
- Reduced tidal volumes
- Intra-abdominal pressure (IAP) of 24 mmHg

a) What is the diagnosis? *(1 mark)*

b) How are intra-abdominal hypertension (IAH) and abdominal compartment syndrome (ACS) defined? *(2 marks)*

c) How can IAP be measured in the ventilated patient? *(2 marks)*

d) What are the surgical causes of a raised IAP in patients on the intensive care unit? *(4 marks)*

e) Describe the effect of IAH on the following systems—respiratory, cardiovascular, renal, gastrointestinal, and central nervous *(5 marks)*

f) What treatment options are available for the management of ACS? *(6 marks)*

Answers

a) What is the diagnosis? *(1 mark)*
- Abdominal compartment syndrome

b) How are intra-abdominal hypertension (IAH) and abdominal compartment syndrome (ACS) defined? *(2 marks)*
- IAH—a sustained or repeated pathological elevation of IAP ≥12 mmHg
- ACS—a sustained IAP >20 mmHg (with or without an abdominal perfusion pressure <60 mmHg) that is associated with new organ dysfunction or failure

c) How can IAP be measured in the ventilated patient? *(2 marks)*
- Direct—needle puncture of the abdominal cavity
- Indirect—via a urinary catheter in the bladder or a balloon-tipped catheter inserted into the stomach

d) What are the surgical causes of a raised IAP in patients on the intensive care unit? *(4 marks)*

(1 mark per cause to a maximum of 4)
- Intra-abdominal or retroperitoneal haemorrhage
- Reduction of a large hernia
- Abdominal closure under excessive tension
- Ileus
- Intra-abdominal leak or collection

e) Describe the effect of IAH on the following systems—respiratory, cardiovascular, renal, gastrointestinal, and central nervous *(5 marks)*
- Respiratory:
  - Reduced lung compliance and thoracic volume
  - Basal atelectasis
  - Parenchymal compression potentially resulting in infection, oedema, and an increased risk of ventilator-associated lung injury
- Cardiovascular:
  - Reduced venous return resulting in a reduced cardiac output
- Renal:
  - Reduced renal perfusion
- Gastrointestinal:
  - Hepatic dysfunction, deterioration in gut function, and loss of gut barrier function
- Central nervous:
  - Increased intracranial pressure

f) What treatment options are available for the management of ACS? *(6 marks)*

- Evacuate intraluminal contents—nasogastric and rectal decompression, prokinetic agents, reduced enteral feeding
- Evacuate intra-abdominal fluid collections—percutaneous or surgical drainage, paracentesis
- Improve abdominal wall compliance—sedation and analgesia, neuromuscular blockade, avoidance of head of bed >30 degrees, removal of restrictive dressings
- Optimize fluid administration—avoidance of excessive fluid resuscitation and a positive fluid balance, fluid removal via diuresis or haemofiltration/ultrafiltration
- Optimize systemic and regional perfusion
- Surgical decompression—strongly considered when IAP >20 mmHg with evidence of organ dysfunction or ischaemia

Further reading

Kirkpatrick AW, Roberts DJ, De Waele J, Jaeschke R, Malbrain ML, De Keulenaer B. Intra-abdominal hypertension and the abdominal compartment syndrome: updated consensus definitions and clinical practice guidelines from the World Society of the Abdominal Compartment Syndrome. *Intensive Care Medicine* 2013;37:1190–1206.

FFICM syllabus references 1.1, 2.1, 2.2, 2.7, 2.8, 3.3, 3.4, 3.7 4.4, 5.17, 5.19, 6.1, 12.2.
CoBaTrICE domains 1, 2, 3, 4, 5, 6.

OSCE 1 station 7—data

Questions

a) What is an ultrasound wave? *(1 mark)*
b) What is the relationship between the velocity, frequency, and wavelength of a sound wave? *(1 mark)*
c) With respect to the use of ultrasound for imaging, what characteristic of the waveform determines the resolution of the image? *(2 marks)*
d) What is the disadvantage of using a short wavelength when using ultrasound for imaging? *(1 mark)*
e) What factors can make transthoracic echocardiography technically difficult in the ventilated patient? *(4 marks)*

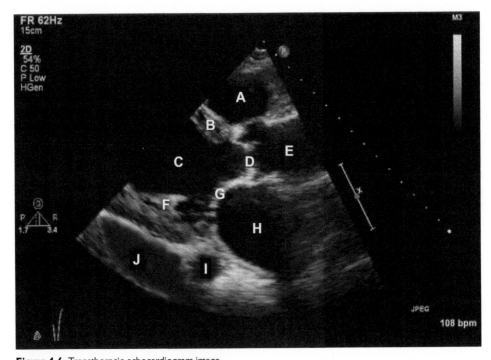

Figure 1.6 Transthoracic echocardiogram image
Reproduced from *Acute and Critical Care Echocardiography*, Colebourn C and Newton J, Figure 6.9. © 2017 Oxford University Press. Reproduced with permission of the Licensor through PLSclear

Look at Figure 1.6.

f) Identify the structures labelled A–I in this parasternal long-axis view *(9 marks)*
g) What is shown in area J? *(1 mark)*
h) How can we determine from this image that the fluid shown in area J is pleural, rather than pericardial? *(1 mark)*

Answers

a) What is an ultrasound wave? *(1 mark)*
  - A sound that is too high a frequency (>20 kHz) to be perceived by the human ear
b) What is the relationship between the velocity, frequency, and wavelength of a sound wave? *(1 mark)*
  - Velocity = wavelength × frequency
c) With respect to the use of ultrasound for imaging, what characteristic of the waveform determines the resolution of the image? *(2 marks)*
  - Wavelength
  - The shorter the wavelength, the higher the resolution
d) What is the disadvantage of using a short wavelength when using ultrasound for imaging? *(1 mark)*
  - The shorter the wavelength, the lower the penetration of the wave
e) What factors can make transthoracic echocardiography particularly difficult in the ventilated patient? *(4 marks)*
  - Position—an ideal position for echocardiography is with the patient lying in the left lateral position, which may be difficult to achieve
  - Devices and monitoring (e.g. electrocardiogram leads, chest drains, dressings) may interfere with probe placement
  - Ventilation—the patient cannot be asked to alter their breathing pattern to aid images (hold their breath etc.)
  - Positive intrathoracic pressure can result in hyperinflated lungs which 'hide' the heart
f) Identify the structures labelled A–I in this parasternal long-axis view *(9 marks)*
  - A—right ventricle
  - B—intraventricular septum
  - C—left ventricle
  - D—aortic valve
  - E—ascending aorta
  - F—papillary muscle
  - G—mitral valve
  - H—left atrium
  - I—descending aorta
g) What is shown in area J? *(1 mark)*
  - A left-sided pleural effusion
h) How can we determine from this image that the fluid shown in area J is pleural, rather than pericardial? *(1 mark)*
  - Pleural fluid tracks behind the descending aorta. Pericardial fluid tracks between the left atrium and the descending aorta

Notes

While the ability to perform echocardiography is not part of the UK syllabus for training in intensive care medicine, the requirement to interpret imaging studies makes some knowledge of anatomy and common findings fair game.

Further reading

E-learning for Healthcare. ICE-BLU. Available at: https://www.e-lfh.org.uk/programmes/icu-echoultrasound [accessed 8 January 2018].

FFICM syllabus references 2.6, 3.3.
CoBaTrICE domain 2.

OSCE 1 station 8—data

Questions

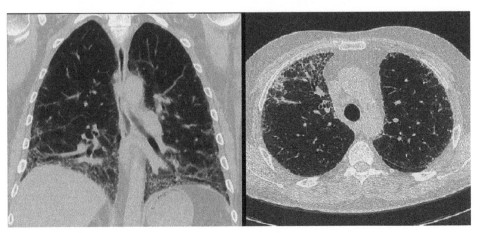

Figure 1.7 HRCT chest
Reproduced from *Challenging Concepts in Respiratory Medicine: Cases with Expert Commentary*, Schomberg, L et al., Figure 10.3.
© 2017 Oxford University Press. Reproduced with permission of the Licensor through PLSclear

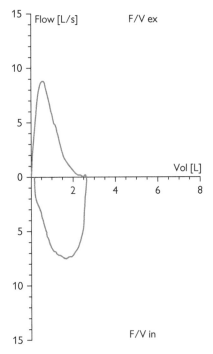

Figure 1.8 Flow–volume loop
Reproduced from *Challenging Concepts in Respiratory Medicine: Cases with Expert Commentary*, Schomberg, L et al., Figure 10.1.
© 2017 Oxford University Press. Reproduced with permission of the Licensor through PLSclear

You are asked to review a 69-year-old man with low oxygen saturations and a 6-month history of progressive breathlessness. Three weeks ago he developed fevers and a cough productive of green sputum. Since admission he has been reviewed by a respiratory physician who requested a high-resolution computed tomography scan (HRCT) and pulmonary function tests.

Look at Figure 1.7.

a) What abnormalities are shown on this HRCT image? *(3 marks)*

Look at Figure 1.8.

b) What category of lung disease is demonstrated by this flow–volume loop? *(1 mark)*
c) Complete Table 1.3q *(3 marks)*

Table 1.3q Pulmonary function tests

Measurement	Value
Forced vital capacity	
Peak inspiratory flow rate	
Peak expiratory flow rate	

The respiratory consultant has written in the notes 'interstitial lung disease, most likely idiopathic pulmonary fibrosis (IPF)'

d) Other than IPF, what are the other potential causes of interstitial lung disease? *(5 marks)*
e) What are the potential causes of a rapid clinical deterioration in patients with IPF? *(5 marks)*
f) What treatment is advocated for acute exacerbations of IPF? *(1 mark)*
g) What is the expected life expectancy for someone diagnosed with IPF? *(1 mark)*
h) What is the predicted mortality for patients with an acute exacerbation of IPF? *(1 mark)*

Answers

a) What abnormalities are shown on this HRCT image? *(3 marks)*
  - Reticular shadowing in a predominantly subpleural distribution
  - Bronchiectasis
  - Honeycombing

b) What category of lung disease is demonstrated by this flow–volume loop? *(1 mark)*
  - Restrictive lung disease

c) Complete Table 1.3a *(3 marks)*

Table 1.3a Pulmonary function tests

Measurement	Value
Forced vital capacity	2.6 L
Peak inspiratory flow rate	7.5 L/second
Peak expiratory flow rate	9 L/second

d) Other than IPF, what are the other potential causes of interstitial lung disease? *(5 marks)*
  - Inhaled substances (e.g. asbestos, silica, beryllium)
  - Drug induced
  - Connective tissue and autoimmune diseases
  - Infection
  - Malignancy

e) What are the potential causes of a rapid clinical deterioration in patients with IPF? *(5 marks)*
  - Infection
  - Pulmonary embolism
  - Pulmonary hypertension leading to heart failure
  - Pneumothorax
  - Acute exacerbation of IPF

f) What treatment is advocated for acute exacerbations of IPF? *(1 mark)*
  - Corticosteroids

g) What is the expected life expectancy for someone diagnosed with IPF? *(1 mark)*
  - 15% 5-year survival, with an average life expectancy of approximately 4 years

h) What is the predicted mortality for patients with an acute exacerbation of IPF? *(1 mark)*
  - 70–80%

Further reading

Raghu G, Collard HR, Egan JJ, Martinez FJ, Behr J, Brown KK, et al. An official ATS/ERS/JRS/ALAT statement: idiopathic pulmonary fibrosis: evidence-based guidelines for diagnosis and management. *American Journal of Respiratory and Critical Care Medicine* 2011;183:788–824.

FFICM syllabus references 1.1, 2.2, 2.6, 2.8, 3.2.
CoBaTrICE domains 1, 2, 3.

OSCE 1 station 9—data

Questions

A 26-year-old woman has presented to the emergency department with abdominal pain and vomiting 2 days after a prolonged period of deliberate paracetamol ingestion. Her paracetamol level is 60 mg/L.

a) What treatment should be started in this patient? *(1 mark)*

b) Which patients do not require treatment following a staggered overdose of paracetamol? *(4 marks)*

c) In which patient groups should a lower threshold for N-acetylcysteine (NAC) be considered than that suggested by a nomogram? *(3 marks)*

d) How does NAC administration reduce hepatotoxicity? *(2 marks)*

e) The patient develops vomiting and urticaria after commencing the NAC infusion. Should the infusion be stopped? *(1 mark)*

f) What can be done to reduce nausea and anaphylactoid reactions when administering NAC? *(2 marks)*

g) What are the three major sources of mortality in liver failure secondary to paracetamol toxicity? *(3 marks)*

h) What are the King's College criteria for liver transplantation in cases of paracetamol toxicity? *(2 marks)*

i) What other biochemical criteria for liver transplantation in cases of paracetamol toxicity are included in the modified King's College criteria? *(2 marks)*

Answers

a) What treatment should be started in this patient? *(1 mark)*
- Intravenous *N*-acetylcysteine via a standardized regimen

b) Which patients do not require treatment following a staggered overdose of paracetamol? *(4 marks)*
- Paracetamol levels are below 10 mg/L *and*
- International normalized ratio (INR) 1.3 or less *and*
- Alanine aminotransferase (ALT) is normal *and*
- The patient has no symptoms of liver damage

c) In which patient groups should a lower threshold for *N*-acetylcysteine (NAC) be considered than that suggested by a nomogram? *(3 marks)*
- Uncertain timing of overdose
- Staggered overdose
- Concurrent overdose of drugs delaying gastric emptying

d) How does NAC administration reduce hepatotoxicity? *(2 marks)*
- By replenishing stores of glutathione
- ... preventing the toxic paracetamol metabolite (*N*-acetyl-*p*-benzoquinone imine) from causing direct hepatocellular toxicity

e) The patient develops vomiting and urticaria after commencing the NAC infusion. Should the infusion be stopped? *(1 mark)*
- The infusion should be continued; anaphylactoid reactions are relatively common and the balance of risk is in favour of continued treatment with NAC

f) What can be done to reduce nausea and anaphylactoid reactions when administering NAC? *(2 marks)*
- Reduce the rate of infusion
- Steroids can be used for severe anaphylactoid reactions

g) What are the three major sources of mortality in liver failure secondary to paracetamol toxicity? *(3 marks)*
- Cerebral oedema
- Infection
- Multiorgan failure

h) What are the King's College criteria for liver transplantation in cases of paracetamol toxicity? *(2 marks)*
- pH <7.3 following volume resuscitation >24 hours post ingestion *or*
- Prothrombin time >100 seconds (INR >6.5), creatinine >300 µmol/L, and grade III/IV encephalopathy within a 24-hour time span

(Reprinted from *Gastroenterology*, 97, 2, O'Grady JG, Alexander GJ, Hayllar KM, and Williams R, Early indicators of prognosis in fulminant hepatic failure, pp. 439–45, Copyright 1989, with permission from Elsevier and the AGA Institute.)

i) What other biochemical criteria for liver transplantation in cases of paracetamol toxicity are included in the modified King's College criteria? *(2 marks)*
- Lactate >3.5 mmol/L after early resuscitation (< 4 hours) *or*
- Lactate >3 mmol/L following full fluid resuscitation (12 hours) or 24 hours post paracetamol ingestion

(Reproduced from *The Lancet*, 359, 9306, Bernal W, Donaldson N, Wyncoll D, and Wendon J, Blood lactate as an early predictor of outcome in paracetamol-induced acute liver failure: a cohort study, pp. 558–63, Copyright 2002, with permission from Elsevier.)

Notes

This question is a reminder to always look for the detail in topics that are clinically very familiar.

Further reading

Medicines and Healthcare products Regulatory Agency. Treating paracetamol overdose with intravenous acetylcysteine: new guidance. 2014. Available at: https://www.gov.uk/drug-safety-update [accessed 26 October 2019].

FFICM syllabus references 2.2, 2.8, 3.1, 3.5.
CoBaTrICE domains 1, 2, 3.

OSCE 1 station 10—data

Questions

You have been asked to review a mountain bike rider in the emergency department who has fallen 6 metres down a rocky embankment at high speed.

The primary survey revealed a patent airway, respiratory rate of 20 breaths per minute, SpO_2 of 95% in air, blood pressure of 82/40 mmHg, heart rate of 58 beats per minute (regular), and a Glasgow Coma Scale score of 15. There are significant facial and chest abrasions.

a) What causes of shock should be considered in this trauma patient? (3 marks)
b) Aside from hypotension and bradycardia, what other clinical signs of spinal cord injury might be present? (3 marks)

A computed tomography (CT) scan of the chest, abdomen, and pelvis ruled out internal haemorrhage. Look at Figure 1.9.

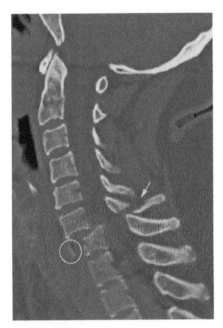

Figure 1.9 Sagittal reconstructed CT scan of the neck

Reproduced from *Musculoskeletal Imaging Volume 1: Trauma, Arthritis, and Tumor and Tumor-Like Conditions*, Mihra S. Taljanovic *et al.*, Figure 2.3. © 2019 Oxford University Press. Reproduced with permission of the Licensor through PLSclear.

c) What abnormalities have been highlighted in this CT image? (2 marks)
d) How can the degree of anterolisthesis be used to differentiate between unilateral and bilateral facet joint dislocation? (1 mark)
e) How should neurogenic shock be managed? (4 marks)
f) Why does bradycardia occur in spinal shock? (1 mark)
g) Other than shock, what other life-threatening complications may occur because of the cervical spine injury? (2 marks)

In view of increasing respiratory difficulty, the patient was intubated and ventilated. He underwent reduction and spinal fixation and after several days was extubated.

h) What potential difficulties might arise if reintubation is required? *(2 marks)*

i) What risk is associated with the administration of suxamethonium after spinal cord injury, and how soon after the injury does this risk occur? *(2 marks)*

Answers

a) What causes of shock should be considered in this trauma patient? *(3 marks)*
- Hypovolaemic (haemorrhagic) shock
- Cardiogenic shock
- Neurogenic shock

b) Aside from hypotension and bradycardia, what other clinical signs of spinal cord injury might be present? *(3 marks)*

(1 mark per answer to a maximum of 3)
- Priapism
- Loss of anal tone
- Sensorimotor level
- Abnormal reflexes
- Diaphragmatic breathing

c) What abnormalities have been highlighted in this CT image? *(2 marks)*
- C6 spinous process fracture (arrow)
- C7 teardrop fracture (oval)

d) How can the degree of anterolisthesis be used to differentiate between unilateral and bilateral facet joint dislocation? *(1 mark)*
- In unilateral dislocation, the degree of subluxation is usually less than 25% of the vertebral body anteroposterior width (grade 1 anterolisthesis).

e) How should neurogenic shock be managed? *(4 marks)*
- Cautious fluid boluses
- Atropine or beta agonists for bradycardia
- Vasopressors to improve spinal cord perfusion pressure
- Immobilization to prevent further injury

f) Why does bradycardia occur in spinal shock? *(1 mark)*
- High thoracic injury causes paralysis of the thoracic sympathetic outflow, resulting in unopposed vagal control of heart rate

g) Other than shock, what other life-threatening complications may occur because of the cervical spine injury? *(2 marks)*
- Diaphragmatic paralysis causing respiratory failure
- Airway obstruction from prevertebral swelling

h) What potential difficulties might arise if reintubation is required? *(2 marks)*
- Difficult intubation due to reduced spinal mobility
- Autonomic instability

i) What risk is associated with the administration of suxamethonium after spinal cord injury, and how soon after the injury does this risk occur? *(2 marks)*
- Life-threatening hyperkalaemia
- 72 hours after spinal cord injury

FFICM syllabus references 1.5, 2.6, 4.4.
CoBaTrICE domains 1, 2, 4.

OSCE 1 station 11—data

Questions

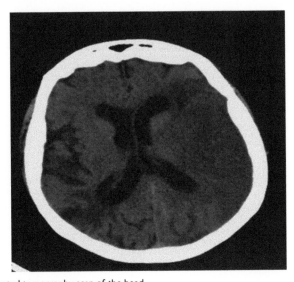

Figure 1.10 Computed tomography scan of the head
Reproduced from *Oxford Textbook of Stroke and Cardiovascular Disease*, Norrving B, Figure 8.1. © 2014 Oxford University Press. Reproduced with permission of the Licensor through PLSclear

Look at Figure 1.10.

a) What is the abnormality? *(1 mark)*
b) Which vascular territory is affected? *(1 mark)*
c) What is the relationship between systolic blood pressure and outcome in acute ischaemic stroke? *(1 mark)*
d) What is the recommendation of the National Institute for Health and Care Excellence (NICE) regarding blood pressure control in the first 24 hours after acute ischaemic stroke? *(2 marks)*
e) What definitive treatment options are available for acute ischaemic stroke? *(2 marks)*
f) What are the eligibility criteria for intravenous thrombolysis in acute stroke? *(2 marks)*
g) What blood pressure targets must be met before thrombolysis can be given in acute stroke? *(2 marks)*
h) Other than patients at risk of bleeding, in which other patient groups might thrombolysis be contraindicated? *(3 marks)*
i) What is the proposed target time from onset of symptoms to endovascular thrombectomy? *(1 mark)*

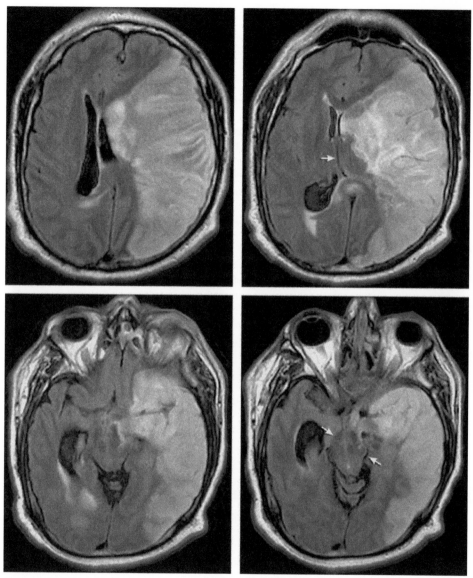

Figure 1.11 MRI of the brain

Reproduced from *The Practice of Emergency and Critical Care Neurology*, Wijdicks EFM, Figure 29.15. Oxford University Press. © 2016 Mayo Foundation for Medical Education and Research. Reproduced with permission of the Licensor through PLSclear

Look at Figure 1.11.

j) What striking abnormalities are seen on this magnetic resonance imaging (MRI) scan and what do the arrows signify? *(2 marks)*

k) What syndrome do these appearances demonstrate? *(1 mark)*

l) What is the evidence for decompressive hemicraniectomy (DH) in malignant middle cerebral artery syndrome? *(2 marks)*

Answers

a) What is the abnormality? *(1 mark)*
    - Acute left-sided cerebral infarction
b) Which vascular territory is affected? *(1 mark)*
    - Left middle cerebral artery (MCA)
c) What is the relationship between systolic blood pressure and outcome in acute ischaemic stroke? *(1 mark)*
    - U-shaped (hypertension is associated with an increased risk of stroke recurrence, whereas hypotension is associated with an increased risk of cardiac events)
d) What is the recommendation of the National Institute for Health and Clinical Excellence (NICE) regarding blood pressure control in the first 24 hours after acute ischaemic stroke? *(2 marks)*
    - NICE guidance does not recommend lowering of blood pressure in this period except:
      - To facilitate thrombolysis
      - In cases of pre-eclampsia/eclampsia, aortic dissection, or hypertensive; encephalopathy, nephropathy, cardiac failure
e) What definitive treatment options are available for acute ischaemic stroke? *(2 marks)*
    - Thrombolysis
    - Endovascular thrombectomy with or without stenting
f) What are the eligibility criteria for intravenous thrombolysis in acute stroke? *(2 marks)*
    - Administration within 4.5 hours of symptom onset
    - Exclusion of acute intracranial haemorrhage
g) What blood pressure targets must be met before thrombolysis can be given in acute stroke? *(2 marks)*
    - Systolic blood pressure <185 mmHg
    - Diastolic blood pressure <110 mmHg
h) Other than patients at risk of bleeding, in which other patient groups might thrombolysis be contraindicated? *(3 marks)*

    (1 mark per contraindication to a maximum of 3)
    - Significant hyperglycaemia/hypoglycaemia
    - Seizure activity at onset of symptoms
    - Rapidly improving symptoms
    - High premorbid dependency or an advanced directive refusing treatment

i) What is the proposed target time from onset of symptoms to endovascular thrombectomy? *(1 mark)*
    - Within 6 hours
j) What striking abnormalities are seen on this MRI scan and what do the arrows signify? *(2 marks)*
    - Large left MCA infarct with mass effect and midline shift
    - Compression of the third ventricle and the brainstem
k) What syndrome do these appearances demonstrate? *(1 mark)*
    - Malignant MCA syndrome
l) What is the evidence for decompressive hemicraniectomy (DH) in malignant middle cerebral artery syndrome? *(2 marks)*

- The HAMLET trial showed that DH within 48 hours was associated with a reduction in mortality and of severe disability. It also demonstrated an increase in functional independence at 6 months
- The DESTINY II trial showed that in patients >60 years old, improved survival was at the expense of severe functional debilitation

Further reading

Evans M, White P, Cowlet P, Werring D. Revolution in acute ischaemic stroke care: a practical guide to mechanical thrombectomy. *Practical Neurology* 2017;17:252–265.

National Institute for Health and Care Excellence (NICE). Stroke and transient ischaemic attack in over 16s: diagnosis and initial management. NICE Clinical Guideline [CG68]. 2017. Available at: https://www.nice.org.uk/guidance/cg68 [accessed 25 November 2017].

FFICM syllabus references 1.3, 2.6, 3.6.
CoBaTrICE domains 2, 3.

OSCE 1 station 12—equipment

Questions

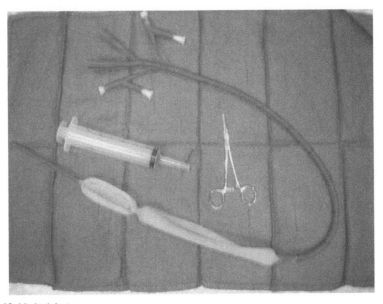

Figure 1.12 Medical device
Reproduced from *Oxford Textbook of Critical Care, Second Edition*, Webb A, et al., Figure 178.2. © 2016 Oxford University Press. Reproduced with permission of the Licensor through PLSclear

Look at Figure 1.12.

a) What is the name of this device? *(1 mark)*

b) What are the differences between the Minnesota tube (MT) and the Sengstaken–Blakemore tube (SBT)? *(2 marks)*

c) What is the indication for the use of a device such as a SBT or MT? *(2 marks)*

d) Outline how you would insert a MT in a patient who is invasively ventilated *(8 marks)*

e) What are the major contraindications to balloon tamponade? *(2 marks)*

f) What are the potential complications of balloon tamponade? *(4 marks)*

g) What is the recommended therapeutic treatment for patients with variceal haemorrhage who continue to bleed despite medical (pharmacological and repeat endoscopic) treatment and balloon tamponade? *(1 mark)*

Answers

a) What is the name of this device? *(1 mark)*
  - Minnesota tube

b) What are the differences between the Minnesota tube (MT) and the Sengstaken–Blakemore tube (SBT)? *(2 marks)*
  - The SBT has three ports, whereas the MT also has an additional port for oesophageal suction
  - The MT has a higher volume gastric balloon (450–500 mL vs 250–300 mL)

c) What is the indication for the use of a device such as a SBT or MT? *(2 marks)*
  - Bleeding upper gastrointestinal varices ...
  - resistant to medical and/or endoscopic treatment

d) Outline how you would insert a MT in a patient who is invasively ventilated *(8 marks)*
  - Test the balloon integrity and record the pressure using a manometer at each volume inflation, 50 mL, 100 mL, 200 mL, etc.
  - Measure from the angle of the mouth to xiphisternum to estimate the depth of insertion
  - Insert under direct vision to at least the estimated length outlined previously via the nose or mouth
  - Inflate the gastric balloon with 25–50 mL of air and X-ray to confirm the gastric balloon is in the stomach
  - Inflate the gastric balloon in increments of 50–100 mL of air (contrast liquid can be used to facilitate imaging as an alternative)
  - Monitor gastric balloon pressure during incremental inflation. If a rise in pressure of more than 15 mmHg above the baseline pressure is seen, suspect oesophageal or duodenal migration and repeat imaging
  - Once the balloon is fully inflated, clamp and withdraw the tube until resistance is felt as it impacts against the gastro-oesophageal junction. Note this depth and attach traction to the device to maintain gentle pressure
  - If bleeding continues, consider inflation of the oesophageal balloon

e) What are the major contraindications to balloon tamponade? *(2 marks)*
  - Oesophageal abnormalities (e.g. stricture, acute rupture, or oesophagectomy)
  - Abnormalities of the proximal upper gastrointestinal tract (e.g. significant hiatus hernia, fundoplication, roux-en-Y)

f) What are the potential complications of balloon tamponade? *(4 marks)*

  (1 mark per complication to a maximum of 4)
  - Migration resulting in viscus perforation, pneumothorax, pneumomediastinum, pneumoperitoneum, or upper airway obstruction
  - Necrosis of the oesophagus or gastro-oesophageal junction
  - Pressure damage at the mouth or nose
  - Aspiration pneumonitis
  - Cardiac arrhythmias

g) What is the recommended therapeutic treatment for patients with variceal haemorrhage who continue to bleed despite medical (pharmacological and repeat endoscopic) treatment and balloon tamponade? *(1 mark)*
  - Placement of a transjugular intrahepatic portosystemic shunt (TIPPS)

Further reading

Stanley AJ, Laine L. Management of acute upper gastrointestinal bleeding. *BMJ* 2019;364:l536.

FFICM syllabus references 3.1, 3.5, 5.18.
CoBaTrICE domains 1, 3, 4, 5.

OSCE 1 station 13—equipment

Questions

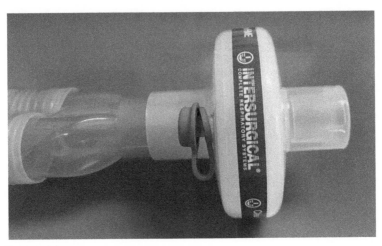

Figure 1.13 Medical device
Reproduced with kind permission from Intersurgical

a) What are the effects on the respiratory system of ventilation using cold, dry gas? *(5 marks)*

Look at Figure 1.13.

b) What is this piece of equipment called? *(1 mark)*
c) In what situations might a heat and moisture exchanger not perform as well as it normally would? *(3 marks)*
d) What are the risks associated with using a heat and moisture exchanger? *(3 marks)*
e) By what name is a heat and moisture exchanger designed for long-term use on a tracheostomy commonly known? *(1 mark)*
f) What is the difference between passive and active humidification? *(1 mark)*
g) When using active humidification, what problems can be caused by condensation in the ventilation circuit tubing? *(3 marks)*
h) How can condensation in the ventilation circuit tubing be avoided when using active humidification? *(3 marks)*

Answers

a) What are the effects on the respiratory system of ventilation using cold, dry gas? *(5 marks)*
  - Mucosal dysfunction
  - Lesions of the epithelium and mucosa
  - Decreased compliance
  - Decreased functional residual capacity
  - Increased energy expenditure

b) What is this piece of equipment called? *(1 mark)*
  - Heat and moisture exchanger (or a hygroscopic condenser humidifier)

c) In what situations might a heat and moisture exchanger not perform as well as it normally would? *(3 marks)*
  - Expired volume much less than inspiratory volume (e.g. large bronchopleural fistulae)
  - Hypothermia
  - High minute ventilation

d) What are the risks associated with using a heat and moisture exchanger? *(3 marks)*
  - Obstruction of the ventilator circuit by secretions, blood, or vomit
  - Increased dead space
  - Increased expiratory resistance

e) By what name is a heat and moisture exchanger designed for long-term use on a tracheostomy commonly known? *(1 mark)*
  - Swedish nose

f) What is the difference between passive and active humidification? *(1 mark)*
  - Active humidification requires a power or water supply, passive requires neither

g) When using active humidification, what problems can be caused by condensation in the ventilation circuit tubing? *(3 marks)*
  - Obstruction of the ventilator circuit
  - Auto-triggering of the ventilator
  - Increased risk of respiratory infection

h) How can condensation in the ventilation circuit tubing be avoided when using active humidification? *(3 marks)*
  - Heating the ventilator circuit distal to the humidifier
  - Adding a heated expiratory filter to the circuit
  - Adding water traps to the circuit

Notes

Humidification is employed on all your ventilated patients but it's not something we usually pay too much attention to! Take a moment at work to look around for other pieces of equipment and topics that are familiar, but you don't know in enough detail to answer a question about.

Further reading

Lei Y. Humidification, nebulization, and gas filtering. In: Lei Y. *Medical Ventilator System Basics: A Clinical Guide*, pp. 61–82. Oxford: Oxford University Press; 2017.

FFICM syllabus references 5.1, 11.4.
CoBaTrICE domains 4, 7.

OSCE 2

OSCE 2 station 1—professionalism

Questions

A patient is being cared for in the emergency department having been intubated and ventilated. A computed tomography scan shows extensive subarachnoid haemorrhage with blood in the ventricular system. The neurosurgical team have given their opinion that the bleed is incompatible with a good functional recovery and that there is no neurosurgical management option. The patient's family have said that the patient would want 'everything to be done' and that they share this view.

You decide that the patient should be admitted to the intensive care unit and go to speak to the nurse in charge. He asks:

a) 'We don't have any beds—how can I admit them?' *(3 marks)*

After your discussion, the nurse is confident he can admit the patient. He does, however, have further questions:

b) 'The neurosurgeons have said this patient isn't going to do well, why should we admit them?' *(3 marks)*
c) 'Are you just admitting for organ donation?' *(2 marks)*
d) 'Are you planning to perform any procedures once the patient arrives?' *(2 marks)*
e) 'How long are you going to continue treatment if there is no change in the patient's condition?' *(1 mark)*
f) 'What will you do if you see an improvement?' *(1 mark)*
g) 'What are you going to tell the family?' *(3 marks)*
h) 'Will you keep going if the family change their mind and don't think this is something he would have wanted?' *(2 marks)*

Answers

a) 'We don't have any beds—how can I admit them?' *(3 marks)*
   - Explore whether any patients are fit for discharge or to step down from level 3 to level 2 care
   - Explore whether there are any other resources within the hospital that can be utilized
   - Explore whether any patients are suitable for transfer to another hospital
b) 'The neurosurgeons have said this patient isn't going to do well, why should we admit them?' *(3 marks)*
   - Acknowledge that a poor outcome is most likely
   - Explain that early prognostication can be imprecise in this patient group
   - Give examples of potential cofounders, e.g. seizure activity, drugs
c) 'Are you just admitting for organ donation?' *(2 marks)*
   - State 'no', and that that the reason for admission is for prognostication
   - Acknowledge that organ donation may be an outcome of admission as a normal part of end of life care
d) 'Are you planning to perform any procedures once the patient arrives?' *(2 marks)*
   - Explain that an arterial line will be required
   - State that a central line may be required for the management of haemodynamic instability
e) 'How long are you going to continue treatment if there is no change in the patient's condition?' *(1 mark)*
   - State that the period of observation will be between 24 and 72 hours
f) 'What will you do if you see an improvement?' *(1 mark)*
   - Explain this will prompt further discussion with the neurosurgeons
g) 'What are you going to tell the family?' *(3 marks)*
   - That death or poor functional recovery is the most likely outcome
   - That more time is required for accurate prognostication
   - That if there is significant deterioration this may represent inevitable death and consideration will be given to the withdrawal of treatment
h) 'Will you keep going if the family change their mind and don't think this is something he would have wanted?' *(2 marks)*

   - State that this would remain a best interests decision, taking into account this new information
   - Explain that if there have been no signs of recovery active treatment would be withdrawn at that time

General communication *(3 marks)*
   Marks awarded for behaviours such as the following:

   - Demonstrates appropriate assertiveness
   - Demonstrates politeness and respectful interaction when addressing concerns
   - Appropriate pace and volume of speech

Further reading

Harvey D, Butler J, Groves J, Manara A, Menon D, Thomas E, et al. Management of perceived devastating brain injury after hospital admission: a consensus statement from stakeholder professional organizations. *British Journal of Anaesthesia*, 2018;120:138–145.

FFICM syllabus references 1.4, 3.6, 7.1, 7.4, 7.5, 8.1, 12.2, 12.4, 12.12
CoBaTrICE domains 3, 8, 12.

OSCE 2 station 2—resuscitation

Questions

You are asked by a nurse to review a patient because of a problem with their temporary percutaneous tracheostomy. The patient is breathing spontaneously, with an assisted mode of ventilation.

a) Outline how you would assess the patient *(7 marks)*

You find that the patient is making respiratory effort. His oxygen saturation is 90%, blood pressure is 160/70 mmHg, and heart rate is 100 beats per minute (normal sinus rhythm).

b) What would your next actions be? *(2 marks)*

You are unable to pass a suction catheter.

c) What would your next actions be? *(2 marks)*

You are still unable to pass a suction catheter, and you notice the patient's saturation is now 85%.

d) What would your next actions be? *(3 marks)*

The patient is making weak respiratory effort. His oxygen saturation is 80%, blood pressure is 152/75 mmHg, and hear rate is 120 beats per minute regular.

e) What would your next actions be? *(3 marks)*

Your assistant asks if you would like the tube cut.

f) Would you? *(2 marks)*

Answers

a) Outline how you would assess the patient (7 marks)
- Call for help
- Confirm breathing by:
  - Looking, listening, and feeling at both the mouth and tracheostomy
  - Attaching a Water's (Mapleson C) circuit to the tracheostomy
  - Looking at the capnography trace
- Apply high-flow oxygen via a facemask
- Apply high-flow oxygen via the tracheostomy
- Ask for vital signs

b) What would your next actions be? (2 marks)
- Remove the inner catheter and speaking valve if in situ
- Check the patency of the tracheostomy tube by attempting to pass a suction catheter

c) What would your next actions be? (2 marks)
- Deflate the cuff of the tracheostomy tube
- Reassess the patency of the tracheostomy tube

d) What would your next actions be? (3 marks)
- Remove the tracheostomy tube
- Reapply oxygen to the stoma site (it should still be in place over the patient's face)
- Reassess the patient

e) What would your next actions be? (3 marks)
- Support respiration via bag–valve mask ventilation of the upper airway
- Cover the stoma
- Prepare for oral reintubation

f) Your assistant asks if you would like the tube cut. Would you? (2 marks)
- No
- You will advance the tube beyond the stoma site

Effective use of the assistant (1 mark)

Notes

The examiners would expect your management of this patient to follow the guidelines produced by the National Tracheostomy Safety Project.

If you efficiently work through a standard treatment algorithm you may well 'complete' the simulation scenarios before the 7-minute period has passed; the scenarios are written to allow enough time for a 'nervous candidate' to reach the end. It is important therefore that you should be efficient but also take your time, so you don't miss the easy marks (such as calling for help, reassessing, or applying oxygen).

Further reading

McGrath BA, Bates L, Atkinson D, Moore JA. Multidisciplinary guidelines for the management of tracheostomy and laryngectomy airway emergencies. *Anaesthesia* 2012;67:1025–1041.

National Tracheostomy Safety Project. Available at: https://www.tracheostomy.org.uk [accessed 8 January 2018].

FFICM syllabus references 2.7, 5.1, 5.2, 5.4, 11.4, 11.6, 12.2
CoBaTrICE domains 2, 5, 11.

OSCE 2 station 3—data

Questions

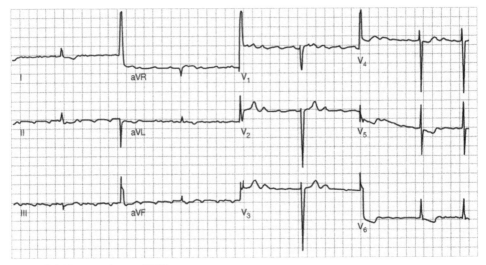

Figure 2.1 Electrocardiogram (ECG)

Reproduced from *Mayo Clinic Cardiology: Concise Textbook, Fourth Edition*, Murphy JG and Lloyd MA, Figure 17.43. Oxford University Press. © 2012 Mayo Foundation for Medical Education and Research. Reproduced with permission of the Licensor through PLSclear

A 78-year-old woman has been admitted to the intensive care unit with hypotension and bradycardia following a 4-day diarrhoeal illness with vomiting. She is in acute renal failure with a serum potassium level of 6.9 mmol/L (normal range: 3.5–5.3 mmol/L). Her medication history is unknown. Her electrocardiogram (ECG) is shown in Figure 2.1.

a) What abnormalities are shown on the ECG? *(4 marks)*
b) What is the most likely cause of the bradycardia? *(1 mark)*

A medication history is obtained, which includes digoxin.

c) How does digoxin improve cardiac contractility? *(2 marks)*
d) How does digoxin cause a reduction in heart rate? *(1 mark)*
e) Other than arrhythmias, what are the symptoms of digoxin toxicity? *(3 marks)*
f) What specific treatment is indicated for her digoxin toxicity? *(1 mark)*
g) What two pieces of information can help calculate the dose of digoxin-specific antibody fragments? *(2 marks)*
h) What adverse effects may occur with or following the use of digoxin-specific antibody fragments? *(4 marks)*
i) Should digoxin levels be monitored during and after treatment? Explain your answer *(2 marks)*

Answers

a) What abnormalities are shown on the ECG? *(4 marks)*
   - Ventricular bradycardia
   - Atrial tachycardia
   - Atrioventricular block
   - Reverse tick ST segment changes

b) What is the most likely cause of her bradycardia? *(1 mark)*
   - Digoxin toxicity (exacerbated by acute renal failure)

c) How does digoxin improve cardiac contractility? *(2 marks)*
   - Inhibition of the sodium–potassium ATPase, resulting in an increased exchange of calcium for sodium
   - The resulting increase in cardiac myocyte intracellular calcium increases contractility

d) How does digoxin cause a reduction in heart rate? *(1 mark)*
   - Enhanced vagal activity resulting in prolonged conduction in the atrioventricular node

e) Other than arrhythmias, what are the symptoms of digoxin toxicity? *(3 marks)*

   (1 mark per answer to a maximum of 3)
   - Lethargy
   - Headache
   - Dizziness
   - Confusion
   - Gastrointestinal symptoms (anorexia, abdominal pain, nausea and vomiting, diarrhoea)
   - Visual disturbances (reduced acuity, xanthopsia, chromatopsia)

f) What specific treatment is indicated for her digoxin toxicity? *(1 mark)*
   - Digoxin-specific antibody fragments

g) What two pieces of information can help calculate the dose of digoxin-specific antibody fragments? *(2 marks)*
   - Patient weight
   - Serum digoxin level

h) What adverse effects can occur with or following the use of digoxin-specific antibody fragments? *(4 marks)*

   (1 mark per answer to a maximum of 4)
   - Allergic reaction
   - Hypokalaemia
   - Rebound toxicity
   - Heart failure
   - Arrhythmias

i) Should digoxin levels be monitored during and after treatment? Explain your answer *(2 marks)*
   - No
   - The assay measures digoxin bound to antibody fragments as well as free digoxin thereby overestimating free digoxin levels

Further reading

BMJ Best Practice. Digoxin overdose. Available at: https://bestpractice.bmj.com [accessed 26 October 2019].

FFICM syllabus references 2.2, 2.3, 3.1, 3.10, 4.1
CoBaTrICE domains 1, 2, 3.

OSCE 2 station 4—data

Questions

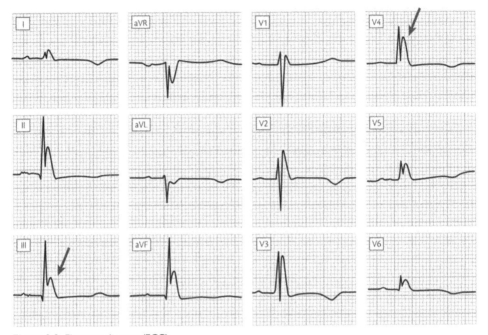

Figure 2.2 Electrocardiogram (ECG)
Reproduced from *The ESC Textbook of Cardiovascular Medicine, Second Edition,* Camm AJ, et al., Figure 2.57. Oxford University Press © 2009 European Society of Cardiology. Reproduced with permission of the Licensor through PLSclear

A 52-year-old man has been brought to the emergency department having been found collapsed next to a canal. He is dressed in multiple layers of cold, wet, and dirty clothing. He has a heart rate of 48 beats per minute and a blood pressure of 88/54 mmHg. His Glasgow Coma Scale score is 9 (E2, M4, V3). The paramedics have been unable to obtain a temperature reading.

Look at the electrocardiogram (ECG) shown in Figure 2.2.

a) What abnormality is marked by the arrows? *(1 mark)*
b) What other abnormalities are seen on this ECG? *(3 marks)*
c) Other than hypothermia, what other causes are there for J waves? *(5 marks)*
d) What are the most reliable sites for measuring temperature in hypothermic patients? *(3 marks)*
e) What central active warming methods are available? *(5 marks)*
f) What changes are made to advanced support algorithms when resuscitating a patient with hypothermia? *(3 marks)*

Answers

a) What abnormality is marked by the arrows? *(1 mark)*
  - Osborne J waves

b) What other abnormalities are seen on this ECG? *(3 marks)*
  - Prolonged PR interval
  - Widened QRS
  - Prolonged QT interval

c) Other than hypothermia, what other causes are there for J waves? *(5 marks)*

(1 mark per cause to a maximum of 5)
  - Hypercalcaemia
  - Brain injury
  - Subarachnoid haemorrhage
  - Vasospastic angina
  - Idiopathic ventricular fibrillation
  - Type 1 Brugada syndrome
  - Normal variant (early repolarization)

d) What are the most reliable sites for measuring temperature in hypothermic patients? *(3 marks)*

(1 mark per site to a maximum of 3)

  - Oesophageal
  - Rectal
  - Bladder
  - Pulmonary artery

e) What central active warming methods are available? *(5 marks)*
  - Warmed humidified inspired gases
  - Warm intravenous fluids
  - Body cavity lavage with warmed fluid (e.g. peritoneal, gastric, bladder, right-sided thoracic lavage)
  - Renal replacement therapy
  - Extracorporeal membrane oxygenation/cardiopulmonary bypass

f) What changes are made to advanced support algorithms when resuscitating a patient with hypothermia? *(3 marks)*
  - No adrenaline or other drugs until patient temperature is >30°C
  - Between 30°C and 35°C, double the dose intervals for advanced life support drugs
  - Shock ventricular fibrillation up to three times if necessary, then no further shocks until the temperature is >30°C

Further reading

Truhlář A, Deakin CD, Soard J, Khalifa GE, Alfonzo A, Bierens JJ, et al. European Resuscitation Council Guidelines for Resuscitation 2015 Section 4. Cardiac arrest in special circumstances. *Resuscitation* 2015;95:148–201.

FFICM syllabus references 1.1, 1.2, 2.3, 3.1, 3.3, 3.6, 4.4, 4.7.
CoBaTrICE domains 1, 2, 4.

OSCE 2 station 5—data

Questions

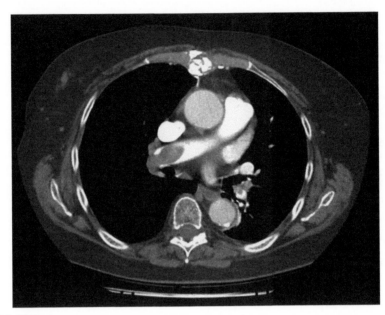

Figure 2.3 CTPA

A 22-year-old man with no significant past medical history has presented with chest pain and dyspnoea 3 days after returning to the UK from Indonesia. The patient has a heart rate of 128 beats per minute and a blood pressure of 118/55 mmHg. A computed tomography pulmonary angiogram (CTPA) is performed and is shown in Figure 2.3.

a) What abnormality is shown on the CTPA image? *(1 mark)*

b) What pharmacological treatment options could be considered in the emergency department? *(3 marks)*

The patient is commenced on low-molecular-weight heparin (LMWH). Eight hours after admission he suddenly develops hypotension.

c) What clinical features would indicate a high risk or massive pulmonary embolism (PE)? *(3 marks)*

d) What is the value of echocardiography when investigating a haemodynamically unstable patient with a suspected high risk or massive PE? *(3 marks)*

Echocardiography shows right ventricular dilatation and pulmonary hypertension.

e) What options are available for treatment of the PE? *(4 marks)*

Systemic thrombolysis is administered, after which there is a significant improvement in the patient's condition. He is commenced on warfarin therapy.

f) When can the LMWH be discontinued? *(2 marks)*

g) How long should this patient remain on warfarin therapy? *(1 mark)*

h) What range of international normalized ratio is considered therapeutic post PE? *(1 mark)*

i) What are the indications for inferior vena cava filter placement after PE? *(2 marks)*

Answers

a) What abnormality is shown on the CTPA image? *(1 mark)*
  - Large filling defect in the right pulmonary artery consistent with pulmonary embolism
b) What pharmacological treatment options could be considered in the emergency department? *(3 marks)*
  - Unfractionated heparin
  - Low-molecular-weight heparin
  - Fondaparinux
c) What clinical features would indicate a high risk or massive pulmonary embolism (PE)? *(3 marks)*
  - Significant hypotension:
    - Blood pressure of <90 mmHg
    - *Or* a drop of >40 mmHg from baseline
  - … not explained by a diagnosis, e.g. arrhythmia, hypovolaemia or sepsis
d) What is the value of echocardiography when investigating a haemodynamically unstable patient with a suspected high risk or massive PE? *(3 marks)*
  - Because it is a bedside test it avoids the risks associated with the transfer of an unstable patient
  - When CTPA is not immediately available, direct visualization of the thrombus, right ventricular dilatation, and pulmonary hypertension may confirm the diagnosis
  - Allows exclusion of other causes of cardiovascular instability, e.g. valvulopathy, left ventricular dysfunction, or pericardial effusion
e) What options are available for treatment of the PE? *(4 marks)*
  - Systemic thrombolysis
  - Surgical embolectomy
  - Catheter-based thrombectomy or thrombolytic techniques
  - Extracorporeal membrane oxygenation
f) When can the LMWH be discontinued? *(2 marks)*
  - After 5 days or …
  - … when the INR remains in the therapeutic range for 24 hours
g) How long should this patient remain on warfarin therapy? *(1 mark)*
  - 3 months
h) What range of international normalized ratio is considered therapeutic post PE? *(1 mark)*
  - 2.0–3.0
i) What are the indications for inferior vena cava filter placement after PE? *(2 marks)*
  - Recurrent thromboembolism despite optimal anticoagulation
  - Contraindication to anticoagulation

Further reading

Konstantinides SV, Torbicki A, Agnelli G, Danchin N, Fitzmaurice D, Galiè N, et al. 2014 European Society of Cardiology Guidelines on the diagnosis and management of acute pulmonary embolism. The Task Force for the Diagnosis and Management of Acute Pulmonary Embolism of the European Society of Cardiology. *European Heart Journal* 2014;35:3033–3080.

FFICM syllabus references 2.6, 2.7, 3.3, 4.1, 4.4, 12.2, 12.11.
CoBaTrICE domains 1, 2, 3, 4.

OSCE 2 station 6—data

Questions

You have been asked to review a 75-year-old man with urinary sepsis. He is alert and orientated with a respiratory rate of 30 breaths per minute, blood pressure of 78/35 mmHg, temperature of 38.5°C, and a heart rate of 110 beats per minute.

a) What is the patient's quick sequential organ failure assessment score (qSOFA) score? *(1 mark)*

b) What is the significance of a high qSOFA score before admission to critical care? *(2 marks)*

c) How useful a prognostic marker is blood lactate compared with the three criteria used in the qSOFA score (conscious level, respiratory rate, and blood pressure)? *(2 marks)*

d) Why is blood lactate omitted from qSOFA score, given its usefulness as a prognostic marker? *(1 mark)*

The patient is admitted to the critical care unit, and after 2 hours develops septic shock.

e) What is the clinical definition of septic shock? *(3 marks)*

f) Where is central venous oxygen saturation (ScvO$_2$) most commonly measured? *(1 mark)*

g) Where is the mixed venous saturation (SvO$_2$) measured? *(1 mark)*

h) In the healthy state, how and why does the oxygen saturation measured in the superior vena cava (SVC) differ from that measured in the pulmonary artery? *(1 mark)*

i) What are the determinants of venous oxygen saturation? *(4 marks)*

This patient's ScvO$_2$ is measured at 86% (normal range: 70–80%).

j) What are the potential causes of a high ScvO$_2$? *(4 marks)*

Answers

a) What is the patient's qSOFA score? *(1 mark)*
- 2 (systolic blood pressure <100 mmHg and respiratory rate >22 breaths per minute)

b) What is the significance of a high qSOFA score before admission to critical care? *(2 marks)*
- Predicts a high risk of death
- Predicts an increased critical care length of stay

c) How useful a prognostic marker is blood lactate compared with the three criteria used in the qSOFA score (conscious level, respiratory rate, and blood pressure)? *(2 marks)*
- As an individual parameter, lactate performs as well as the other components of qSOFA
- Lactate may also increase the ability of qSOFA to predict mortality

d) Why is blood lactate omitted from qSOFA score, given its usefulness as a prognostic marker? *(1 mark)*
- Not all healthcare systems have immediate access to lactate testing

e) What is the clinical definition of septic shock? *(3 marks)*
- Hypotension requiring vasopressors to maintain a mean arterial pressure ≥65 mmHg
- ... and lactate ≥2 mmol/L
- ... in the absence of hypovolaemia

f) Where is central venous oxygen saturation ($ScvO_2$) most commonly measured? *(1 mark)*
- Superior vena cava

g) Where is the mixed venous saturation (SvO_2) measured? *(1 mark)*
- Pulmonary artery

h) In the healthy state, how and why does the oxygen saturation measured in the superior vena cava (SVC) differ from that measured in the pulmonary artery (PA)? *(1 mark)*
- Saturations in the SVC are generally higher than in the PA, due to the addition of blood from the coronary sinus and the inferior vena cava

i) What are the determinants of venous oxygen saturation? *(4 marks)*
- Arterial oxygen saturation
- Oxygen consumption
- Cardiac output
- Haemoglobin concentration

j) What are the potential causes of a high $ScvO_2$? *(4 marks)*

(1 mark per cause to a maximum of 4)

- Increased cardiac output, e.g. sepsis, hypermetabolic states, inotropes
- Arteriovenous shunting, e.g. sepsis, vasodilators
- Reduced oxygen demand, e.g. hypothermia, sedation, mechanical ventilation
- Left-to-right shunting
- Mitochondrial dysfunction, e.g. sepsis, poisoning
- Blood transfusion

Notes

This question highlights the importance of being able to recall key definitions for conditions that you commonly see.

Further reading

Singer M, Deutschman CS, Seymour CW, Shankar-Hari M, Annane D, Bauer M, et al. The Third International Consensus Definitions for Sepsis and Septic Shock (Sepsis-3). *JAMA* 2016;315:801–810.

FFICM syllabus references 2.7, 3.9.
CoBaTrICE domain 2.

OSCE 2 station 7—data

Questions

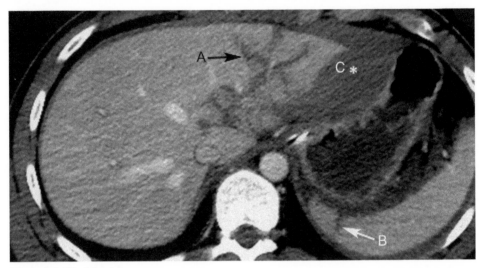

Figure 2.4 CT of the abdomen

Reproduced from *Gastrointestinal Imaging*, Levy AD, Mortele KJ, and and Yeh BM Figure 67.1. © 2015 Oxford University Press. Reproduced with permission of the Licensor through PLSclear

Figure 2.4 is a computed tomography (CT) image from a patient who has been involved in a road traffic accident.

a) What are shown at points A, B, and C? *(3 marks)*

b) Why does traumatic injury more commonly affect the right lobe of the liver? *(3 marks)*

c) In acute traumatic hepatic injury, what features would indicate the need for intervention? *(4 marks)*

The patient underwent an open splenectomy and packing of the liver.

d) What other treatment options are available for management of splenic injury? *(4 marks)*

e) When should this patient receive vaccination after splenectomy, and what vaccinations should be given? *(2 marks)*

f) Which patients should be offered lifelong oral antibiotic prophylaxis post splenectomy? *(4 marks)*

Answers

a) What are shown at points A, B, and C? *(3 marks)*

    A—liver laceration

    B—splenic laceration

    C—haemoperitoneum

b) Why does traumatic injury more commonly affect the right lobe of the liver? *(3 marks)*

- The right lobe is larger
- Rib fractures are more likely to damage the underlying right lobe
- The coronal ligaments insert to the right lobe, therefore shear forces are concentrated on the right lobe

c) In acute traumatic hepatic injury, what features would indicate the need for intervention? *(4 marks)*

- Haemodynamic instability
- Presence of a sentinel clot on CT
- Active extravasation of contrast on CT
- High score on the liver injury scale (3+)

d) What other options are available for the management of splenic injury? *(4 marks)*

- Conservative management
- Angioembolization
- Laparoscopic splenectomy
- Splenic salvage surgery

e) When should this patient receive vaccination after splenectomy, and what vaccinations should be given? *(2 marks)*

- Haemophilus influenzae type b, pneumococcal, and meningococcal 2 weeks post splenectomy
- Influenzae ≥2 weeks post splenectomy, during the vaccination period

f) Which patients should be offered lifelong oral antibiotic prophylaxis post splenectomy? *(4 marks)*

- Age <16 years or >50 years
- Inadequate serological response to pneumococcal vaccination
- History of previous invasive pneumococcal disease
- Patients undergoing splenectomy for haematological malignancy

Further reading

Federico Coccolini F, Montori G, Catena F, Di Saverio S, Biffl W, Moore EE, et al. Liver trauma: WSES position paper. *World Journal of Emergency Surgery* 2015;10:39. Available at: https://wjes.biomedcentral.com/articles/10.1186/s13017-015-0030-9 [accessed 26 February 2018].

FFICM syllabus references 1.5, 2.6, 3.3, 4.2, 6.1.
CoBaTrICE domains 2, 3, 6.

OSCE 2 station 8—data

Questions

You are asked to review a patient who underwent endovascular coiling a week ago following a subarachnoid haemorrhage. Over the last 2 hours the patient, who is not requiring any organ support, has become drowsy.

On examination you find:

- Pulse 65 beats per minute, blood pressure 120/75 mmHg, SaO_2 99% (FiO_2 0.21)
- Glasgow Coma Scale score = E3, M5, V4. Pupillary examination normal. No localizing neurological signs or seizure activity
- Blood glucose 6.8 mmol/L, temperature 36.8°C

A computed tomography scan is also performed, showing no rebleeding, infarction, or hydrocephalus.

a) What are the most likely neurological differential diagnoses? *(3 marks)*

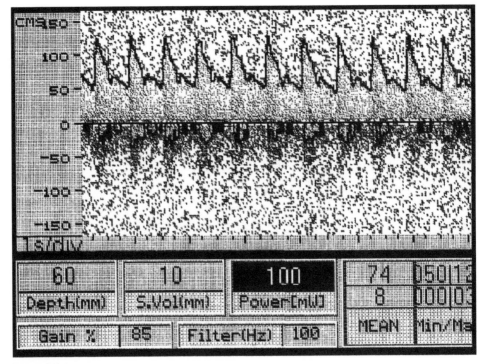

Figure 2.5 Investigation

Reproduced from *The Practice of Emergency and Critical Care Neurology*, Wijdicks EFM, Figure 24.6a. Oxford University Press. © 2016 Mayo Foundation for Medical Education and Research. Reproduced with permission of the Licensor through PLSclear

Look at Figure 2.5.

b) What is this investigation? *(1 mark)*
c) Describe the Doppler effect *(1 mark)*
d) How can transcranial Doppler studies be used to diagnose vasospasm? *(1 mark)*

e) What is the Lindegaard ratio, and how is it useful in the diagnosis of vasospasm? *(2 marks)*
f) When after a subarachnoid haemorrhage are patients at the greatest risk of vasospasm? *(1 mark)*
g) What are the risk factors for vasospasm post subarachnoid haemorrhage? *(2 marks)*
h) What strategies are used to prevent vasospasm? *(6 marks)*
i) How is vasospasm treated? *(3 marks)*

Answers

a) What are the most likely neurological differential diagnoses? *(3 marks)*
- Cerebral vasospasm
- Delayed cerebral ischaemia due to local hypoperfusion or disordered autoregulation
- Non-convulsive seizures

b) What is this investigation? *(1 mark)*
- Transcranial Doppler study

c) Describe the Doppler effect *(1 mark)*
- When a sound wave strikes a moving object, the reflected wave undergoes a change in frequency proportional to the velocity of the object. An increase in frequency of a signal is observed when the signal source approaches the observer, and a decrease when moving away

d) How can transcranial Doppler studies be used to diagnose vasospasm? *(1 mark)*
- Vasospasm develops due to a narrowing of the intracranial arteries causing a reduction in blood flow and an increase in mean blood velocity (Bernoulli's law). Doppler studies measure this increased velocity of blood flow

e) What is the Lindegaard ratio, and how is it useful in the diagnosis of vasospasm? *(2 marks)*
- The ratio of the blood velocity in the middle cerebral artery to the velocity in the ipsilateral extracranial portion of the internal carotid artery
- The ratio helps to distinguish hyperaemia from vasospasm. A ratio <3 is suggestive of hyperaemia, >3 suggests mild to moderate vasospasm, and >6 suggests severe vasospasm

f) When after a subarachnoid haemorrhage are patients at the greatest risk of vasospasm? *(1 mark)*
- Days 3–14 post bleed (peak incidence on days 7–8)

g) What are the risk factors for vasospasm post subarachnoid haemorrhage *(2 marks)*

(1 mark per risk factor to a maximum of 2)
- Smoking history
- Hypertension
- Altered mental status at presentation
- Greater intracranial blood volume (higher modified Fischer score)
- Cocaine use

h) What strategies are used to prevent vasospasm? *(6 marks)*
- Supportive care, avoiding:
  - Hypovolaemia
  - Hypotension
  - Hypoxia
  - Hyperthermia (>37.5°C)
- Pharmacological:
  - Calcium channel antagonists—nimodipine
  - Statins

i) How is vasospasm treated? *(3 marks)*
- Euvolaemia
- Induced hypertension, guided by symptom resolution or radiological/sonographic studies (once the aneurysm is protected)
- Endovascular rescue therapy
  - Intra-arterial vasodilators
  - Angioplasty

Notes

The use of 'triple H' therapy (hypervolaemia, hypertension, and haemodilution) has become less common, with recent reviews suggesting a lack of benefit in the prevention of vasospasm and an increased incidence of adverse events related to hypervolaemia. Triple H therapy also has a weak evidence base for the treatment of vasospasm. The evidence base supporting the use of statins for prevention of vasospasm is also poor but given the low-risk profile, statins are commonly used.

Further reading

Lee Y, Zuckerman SL, Mocco J. Current controversies in the prediction, diagnosis and management of cerebral vasospasm: where do we stand? *Neurology Research International* 2013;2013;373458.

Naqvi J, Yap KH, Ahmad G, Ghosh J. Transcranial Doppler ultrasound: a review of the principles and major applications in critical care. *International Journal of Vascular Medicine* 2013;2013:629378.

FFICM syllabus references 1.1, 2.7, 2.8, 3.1, 3.6, 4.1, 4.4, 6.1.
CoBaTrICE domains 2, 3, 4.

OSCE 2 station 9—data

Questions

a) What are the principal uses of capnography within critical care? *(3 marks)*

b) What method of measuring the partial pressure of carbon dioxide is used most commonly in critical care? *(1 mark)*

c) How can the absorption of infrared light be used to measure the partial pressure of carbon dioxide in a gas mixture? *(2 marks)*

d) What are the two types of infrared capnographs? *(2 marks)*

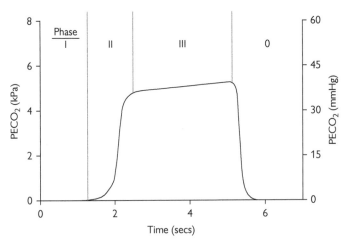

Figure 2.6 Capnography waveform

Reproduced from *Oxford Textbook of Critical Care, Second Edition*, Webb A, et al., Figure 73.1. © 2016 Oxford University Press. Reproduced with permission of the Licensor through PLSclear.

Look at Figure 2.6.

e) What do each of the four phases of the capnography waveform represent? *(4 marks)*

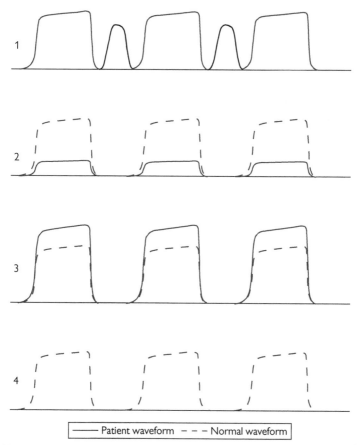

Figure 2.7 Abnormal capnography waveforms

Look at Figure 2.7.

f) Complete Table 2.1q by providing a possible clinical scenario to explain each abnormal capnography waveform *(4 marks)*

Table 2.1q Capnograph abnormalities

Capnograph abnormality	Clinical scenario
Trace 1	
Trace 2	
Trace 3	
Trace 4	

g) What is the expected difference between the end-tidal and arterial partial pressure of carbon dioxide, and what explains this difference? *(2 marks)*

h) Which two groups of patients have a reduced gap between arterial and end-tidal carbon dioxide levels? *(2 marks)*

Answers

a) What are the principal uses of capnography within critical care? *(3 marks)*

(1 mark per use to a maximum of 3)
- Confirmation of tracheal tube placement
- Confirmation of the presence and adequacy of ventilation
- Identification of low cardiac output states
- Identification of bronchospasm

b) What method of measuring the partial pressure of carbon dioxide is used most commonly in critical care? *(1 mark)*
- Infrared spectrography

c) How can the absorption of infrared light be used to measure the partial pressure of carbon dioxide in a gas mixture? *(2 marks)*
- The absorption of infrared light at the wavelength of 4.3 μm is proportional to the concentration of carbon dioxide molecules (Beer's law)
- By measuring the degree of absorption and comparing it with reference tables, the partial pressure can be determined

d) What are the two types of infrared capnographs? *(2 marks)*
- Main stream analysers
- Side stream analysers

e) What do each of the four phases of the capnography waveform represent? *(4 marks)*
- Phase I represents the expiration of carbon dioxide free gas from the anatomical dead space
- Phase II represents mixed gas from airways and alveoli
- Phase III represents gas leaving the alveoli, rising slightly due to variable mixing and time constants
- Phase 0 represents the absence of carbon dioxide during inspiration

f) Complete Table 2.1a by providing a possible clinical scenario to explain each abnormal capnography waveform *(4 marks)*

(1 mark for each correct answer, maximum 1 mark per trace)

Table 2.1a Capnograph abnormalities

Capnograph abnormality	Clinical scenario
Trace 1	Unsynchronized spontaneous respiratory effort
Trace 2	Hyperventilation, hypothermia, low cardiac output, pulmonary embolus
Trace 3	Hypoventilation, hypermetabolic states
Trace 4	Oesophageal intubation, disconnection, apnoea, total airway obstruction, cardiac arrest without resuscitation

g) What is the expected difference between the end-tidal and arterial partial pressure of carbon dioxide, and what explains this difference? *(2 marks)*
- End-tidal partial pressure of carbon dioxide is typically 2–5 mmHg lower than the arterial value
- The difference is caused by the effect of alveolar dead space ventilation on the expired gas mixture

h) Which two groups of patients have a reduced gap between arterial and end-tidal carbon dioxide levels? *(2 marks)*
- Children
- Pregnant women

Further reading

Waldmann C, Rhodes A, Soni N, Handy J. *Oxford Desk Reference: Critical Care*, 2nd Edition. Oxford: Oxford University Press; 2008.

FFICM syllabus references 1.1, 1.2, 1.3, 2.7, 3.8
CoBaTrICE domains 1, 2, 3.

OSCE 2 station 10—data

Questions

A 70-year-old man has oliguria 6 hours after emergency surgery for a leaking abdominal aortic aneurysm.

An arterial blood gas test shows (normal ranges in brackets):

- pH 7.08 (7.35–7.45)
- PCO$_2$ 5.9 kPa (4.7–6.0 kPa)
- PaO$_2$ 13.5 kPa (>10.6 kPa)
- Base excess –12 mmol/L (+/– 2 mmol/L)

Serum potassium is 6.5 mmol/L (3.5–5.3 mmol/L), urea 15 mmol/L (2.5–6.7 mmol/L), and creatinine 300 μmol/L (70–100 μmol/L).

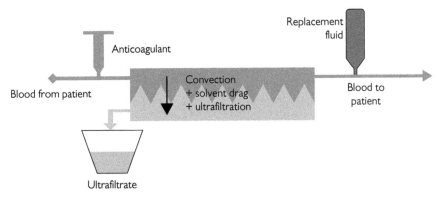

Figure 2.8 Renal replacement therapy

Reproduced from *Oxford Handbook of Critical Care*, Third Edition, Singer M and Webb A, Figure 4.1. © 2009 Oxford University Press. Reproduced with permission of the Licensor through PLSclear.

a) What are the indications for emergency renal replacement therapy? *(5 marks)*

The patient is commenced on renal replacement therapy.

b) What type of renal replacement therapy is shown in Figure 2.8? *(1 mark)*

c) What would be the most significant advantage of changing the circuit so that fluid is replaced before the haemofilter (pre-dilution)? *(1 mark)*

d) With respect to continuous haemofiltration, what is the meaning of the term 'dose'? *(1 mark)*

Despite 4 hours of therapy, the acidaemia does not improve.

e) Why might the acidaemia not improve? *(6 marks)*

f) What medications are used as first-line anticoagulants during continuous haemofiltration? *(4 marks)*

g) What are the risk factors for citrate toxicity during renal replacement therapy with regional citrate anticoagulation? *(2 marks)*

Answers

a) What are the indications for emergency renal replacement therapy? *(5 marks)*
   - Severe metabolic acidaemia
   - Symptomatic uraemia
   - Symptomatic fluid overload resistant to medical management
   - Severe electrolyte derangement resistant to medical management
   - Selected cases of poisoning

b) What type of renal replacement therapy is shown in Figure 2.8? *(1 mark)*
   - Continuous haemofiltration

c) What would be the most significant advantage of changing the circuit so that fluid is replaced before the haemofilter (pre-dilution)? *(1 mark)*
   - Prolonged filter lifespan

d) With respect to continuous haemofiltration, what is the meaning of the term 'dose'? *(1 mark)*
   - The volume of blood 'purified' per unit time

e) Why might the acidaemia not improve? *(6 marks)*

   (1 mark per explanation to a maximum of 6)

   - Low access pressures (e.g. catheter poorly sited, hypovolaemia)
   - High outflow pressures (e.g. patient movement, coughing, obstructed catheter)
   - Interrupted treatment (e.g. circuit clotting or disconnection for transfer)
   - Inadequate prescription
   - Increased demands (patient deterioration)
   - Operator error
   - Mechanical malfunction
   - Filter exhaustion

f) What medications are used as first-line anticoagulants during continuous haemofiltration? *(4 marks)*
   - Citrate
   - Unfractionated heparin
   - Low-molecular-weight heparin
   - Prostacyclin

g) What are the risk factors for citrate toxicity during renal replacement therapy with regional citrate anticoagulation? *(2 marks)*

   (1 mark per risk factor to a maximum of 2)
   - Hepatic dysfunction
   - Low cardiac output
   - Hypocalcaemia
   - Hypoalbuminaemia
   - Hypothermia

Further reading

Gemmell L, Docking R, Black, E. Renal replacement therapy in critical care. *BJA Education* 2017;17:88–93.

FFICM syllabus references 1.1, 2.5, 3.4, 4.7, 4.8, 6.1.
CoBaTrICE domains 2, 4.

OSCE 2 station 11—data

Questions

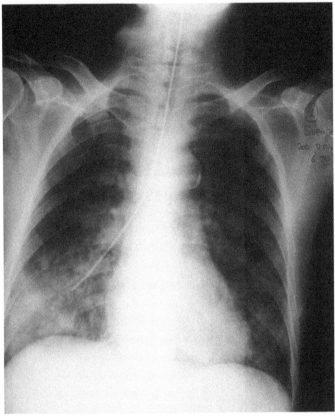

Figure 2.9 Chest X-ray

Reproduced from *Practical Procedures in Anaesthesia and Critical Care*, Jackson G, Soni N, and Whiten C, Figure 6.3. © 2010, Oxford University Press. Reproduced with permission of the Licensor through PLSclear

A 45-year-old man with myasthenia gravis and respiratory failure has been admitted to the intensive care unit. The patient's admission chest X-ray is shown in Figure 2.9.

a) What abnormalities are shown on the chest X-ray? *(2 marks)*
b) What factors can contribute to incorrect nasogastric (NG) tube placement? *(4 marks)*
c) What are the first- and second-line checks for confirmation of NG tube placement? *(2 marks)*
d) What stipulations have been made by NHS Improvement (NHSI) on equipment used for checking the pH of NG tube aspirate? *(3 marks)*
e) What pH range is defined by NHSI as indicative of gastric aspirate? *(1 mark)*
f) Describe how to perform a nose–ear–xiphisternum (NEX) measurement *(3 marks)*
g) What questions should be asked when confirming the correct position of a NG tube on a chest X-ray? *(5 marks)*

Answers

a) What abnormalities are shown on the chest X-ray? *(2 marks)*
   - Right basal consolidation
   - Misplaced endobronchial nasogastric tube

b) What factors can contribute to incorrect nasogastric (NG) tube placement? *(4 marks)*

   (1 mark per factor to a maximum of 4)
   - Lack of corporate quality control (e.g. staff training and competence, awareness of policies, documentation practices)
   - Human factors
   - Patient factors (e.g. absence of cough reflex, poor swallowing reflex)
   - Negligence
   - Procedural factors (e.g. incorrect tube selection, incorrect checking procedures)

c) What are the first- and second-line checks for confirmation of NG tube placement? *(2 marks)*
   - pH testing of gastric aspirate
   - Chest X-ray

d) What stipulations have been made by NHS Improvement (NHSI) on equipment used for checking the pH of NG tube aspirate? *(3 marks)*
   - Litmus paper must not be used
   - pH strips must be CE marked
   - Strips must be intended by the manufacturer to test human gastric aspirate

e) What pH range is defined by NHSI as indicative of gastric aspirate? *(1 mark)*
   - 1–5.5

f) Describe how to perform a nose–ear–xiphisternum (NEX) measurement *(3 marks)*
   - Place the exit port of the NG tube at the tip of the nose
   - Extend the length of the tube to one of the earlobes
   - Holding the tube at the earlobe, extend the remaining length of the NG tube to the lower tip of the xiphisternum and record the length in centimetres

g) What questions should be asked when confirming the correct position of a NG tube on a chest X-ray? *(5 marks)*
   - Is this the most recent chest X-ray of the correct patient?
   - Does the tube follow the contours of the oesophagus and avoid those of the bronchi?
   - Does the tube bisect the carina or bronchi?
   - Does the tube cross the diaphragm in the midline?
   - Is the tip clearly visible below the left hemidiaphragm?

Further reading

NHS Improvement. Patient Safety Alert: Nasogastric tube misplacement: continuing risk of death and severe harm. 2016. Available at: https://www.england.nhs.uk/publication/patient-safety-alert-nasogastric-tube-misplacement-continuing-risk-of-death-and-severe-harm/ [accessed 26 October 2019].

FFICM syllabus references 2.6, 4.9, 5.19, 11.3, 11.4, 11.6, 12.11
CoBaTrICE domains 2, 5, 11, 12.

OSCE 2 station 12—equipment

Questions

a) Why are arterial lines useful in the critical care unit? *(4 marks)*

b) What are the potential causes of a damped arterial pressure waveform? *(4 marks)*

c) Which crystalloids should not be used as arterial line flush fluid and why? *(2 marks)*

d) As well as a reduced systolic pressure, what other changes are seen in the arterial waveform of a patient with peripheral vasodilatation? *(3 marks)*

e) During the administration of antibiotics, a patient with a radial arterial line complains of a sudden onset of severe hand pain. What is the most likely cause? *(1 mark)*

f) What pharmacological agents have been used to maintain distal perfusion after accidental arterial injection of a drug? *(3 marks)*

g) How can the risk of intra-arterial injection be reduced? *(3 marks)*

Answers

a) Why are arterial lines useful in the critical care unit? *(4 marks)*

(1 mark per use to a maximum of 4)
- To allow frequent blood sampling
- To detect haemodynamic instability
- To avoid the tissue damage and discomfort associated with frequent, repeated, non-invasive measurement
- To allow accurate blood pressure measurement in situations such as arrhythmias, obesity, and hypotension
- To allow the use of invasive cardiac output monitoring

b) What are the potential causes of a damped arterial pressure waveform? *(4 marks)*

(1 mark per cause to a maximum of 4)
- Narrow tubing
- Air bubbles
- Kinked tubing
- Arterial spasm
- Blood clot in line
- Reduced flush bag pressure
- Overly compliant tubing

c) Which crystalloids should not be used as arterial line flush fluid and why? *(2 marks)*
- Dextrose-containing solutions
- Risk of pseudohyperglycaemia and subsequent treatment with insulin causing hypoglycaemia

d) As well as a reduced systolic pressure, what other changes are seen in the arterial waveform of a patient with peripheral vasodilatation? *(3 marks)*
- Wide pulse pressure
- Reduced diastolic pressure
- Delayed dicrotic notch

e) During the administration of antibiotics, a patient with a radial arterial line complains of a sudden onset of severe hand pain. What is the most likely cause? *(1 mark)*
- Intra-arterial injection of antibiotic

f) What drugs have been used to maintain distal perfusion after accidental arterial injection of a drug? *(3 marks)*

(1 mark per drug to a maximum of 3)
- Heparin
- Steroids
- Non-steroidal anti-inflammatory drugs
- Local anaesthetic (either intra-arterial or via regional blockage)
- Prostacyclin
- Calcium channel blockers
- Dextran
- Intra-arterial thrombolysis

g) How can the risk of intra-arterial injection be reduced? *(3 marks)*

(1 mark per answer to a maximum of 3)
- Training and education
- Keeping tubing and lines visible
- Removal of unnecessary three-way taps
- Use of colour coded/labelled tubing and three-way taps
- Ensuring that the arterial line is as remote as possible from venous lines

FFICM syllabus references 2.7, 4.1, 5.8, 11.4.
CoBaTrICE domains 2, 5, 11.

OSCE 2 station 13—equipment

Questions

a) What are the indications for a tracheostomy in critical care? *(4 marks)*
b) How do you select the appropriate size of tracheostomy tube? *(2 marks)*
c) How often should the tracheostomy cuff pressure be measured? *(1 mark)*
d) What is the recommended maximum tracheostomy cuff pressure? *(1 mark)*
e) In a patient with a well-established stoma, how frequently should a tracheostomy tube with an inner cannula be changed? *(1 mark)*

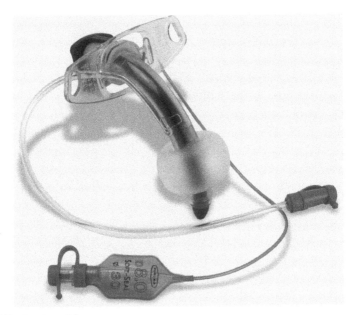

Figure 2.10 Tracheostomy tube
Reproduced with kind permission from Smiths Medical

Look at Figure 2.10.

f) What type of tracheostomy tube is this? *(1 mark)*
g) What are the benefits of a subglottic suction port? *(2 marks)*

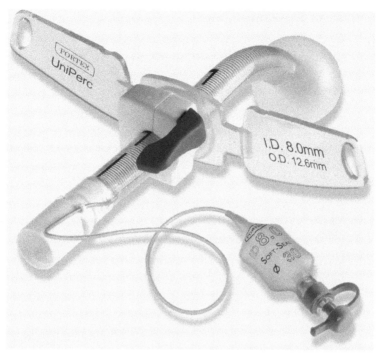

Figure 2.11 Tracheostomy tube
Reproduced with kind permission from Smiths Medical

Look at Figure 2.11.

h) What type of tracheostomy tube is this? *(1 mark)*

i) Which patient groups benefit from the use of a tube with an adjustable flange? *(3 marks)*

j) What were the conclusions of the 'TracMan' study with regard to early versus late tracheostomy insertion? *(4 marks)*

Answers

a) What are the indications for a tracheostomy in critical care? *(4 marks)*
- Upper airway obstruction
- Airway protection
- To facilitate weaning from mechanical ventilation
- To facilitate respiratory secretion management

b) How do you select the appropriate size of tracheostomy tube? *(2 marks)*
- The external diameter should not exceed ¾ of the internal diameter of the tracheal lumen
- The functional internal diameter should be large enough to avoid increased airway resistance and work of breathing

c) How often should the tracheostomy cuff pressure be measured? *(1 mark)*
- 8-hourly

d) What is the recommended maximum tracheostomy cuff pressure? *(1 mark)*
- 25 cmH$_2$O

e) In a patient with a well-established stoma, how frequently should a tracheostomy tube with an inner cannula be changed? *(1 mark)*
- Every 30 days

f) What type of tracheostomy tube is this? *(1 mark)*
- Cuffed tracheostomy with subglottic suction port

g) What are the benefits of a subglottic suction port? *(2 marks)*
- Clearance of oropharyngeal secretions from the proximal trachea reduces ventilator-associated pneumonia
- Insufflating air via the subglottic suction port allows phonation

h) What type of tracheostomy tube is this? *(1 mark)*
- Adjustable flange tracheostomy with inner cannula

i) Which patient groups benefit from the use of a tube with an adjustable flange? *(3 marks)*
- Obese patients with a large neck
- Anatomical abnormalities, e.g. mediastinal masses or burns where the distance to the trachea is increased
- Low-lying tracheostomy stomas

j) What were the conclusions of the 'TracMan' study with regard to early versus late tracheostomy insertion? *(4 marks)*

- No difference in mortality
- No effect on in critical care length of stay
- No effect on hospital length of stay
- Reduction in sedation with early tracheostomy

Notes

If you are asked about research findings, you'll only be asked about the main conclusions of key papers. It would be worth being familiar with these trials and what their main conclusions were.

Further reading

The Intensive Care Society. *Standards for the care of adult patients with a temporary tracheostomy.* London: The Intensive Care Society; 2014. Available at: http://www.ics.ac.uk/ICS/Guidelines [accessed 9 December 2018].

Young D, Harrison DA, Cuthbertson BH, Rowan K, TracMan Collaborators. Effect of early vs late tracheostomy placement on survival in patients receiving mechanical ventilation: the TracMan randomized trial. *JAMA* 2013;309:2121–2129.

FFICM syllabus references 4.6, 5.6, 11.4.
CoBaTrICE domains 3, 5, 11.

OSCE 3

OSCE 3 station 1—professionalism

Questions

A medical student has asked you to teach them how to take blood. You have a dummy arm available.

a) Other than the dummy arm, what other equipment do you need? *(6 marks)*
b) What steps would you take to teach the student? *(8 marks)*

The student asks you how they should best record the learning episode.

c) What would you suggest? *(2 marks)*
d) What are the main benefits of workplace-based assessment? *(4 marks)*

Answers

a) Other than the dummy arm, what other equipment do you need? *(6 marks)*
   - Gloves
   - Needle and blood collection system
   - Sharps bin
   - Tourniquet
   - Antibacterial wipe
   - Dressing

b) What steps would you take to teach the student? *(8 marks)*
   - Establish the student's level of experience
   - Explain how to perform the procedure (including preparation and consent)
   - Demonstrate the procedure
   - Provide encouragement
   - Provide constructive feedback
   - Ask if the student has any questions
   - Provide a summary
   - Plan for further learning

c) What would you suggest? *(2 marks)*

   (1 mark per suggestion to a maximum of 2)
   - A workplace-based assessment such as a direct observation of clinical stills assessment
   - Recording activity in a logbook of procedures
   - Incorporating the event into a personal development plan or learning needs analysis

d) What are the main benefits of workplace-based assessment? *(4 marks)*

   (1 mark per advantage to a maximum of 4)
   - The learner takes ownership of the assessment, promoting active learning
   - The assessment has high construct and content validity
   - The assessment is timely
   - The assessment is structured
   - The assessment is formative, promoting future learning and development

FFICM syllabus references 12.2, 12.10, 12.14.
CoBaTrICE domain 12.

OSCE 3 station 2—resuscitation

Questions

You have been asked to see a patient who has recently been admitted to the high dependency unit following an elective open aortic aneurysm repair.

Despite a continuous epidural infusion and having been given additional epidural boluses totalling 50 mL of 0.25% L-bupivacaine over the last hour, the patient is in pain and has no block to cold. The nursing staff report that the patient is also complaining of 'tingling in his lips' and that he appears 'agitated'. A recent arterial blood gas analysis was unremarkable, and a recent capillary blood sugar test was normal.

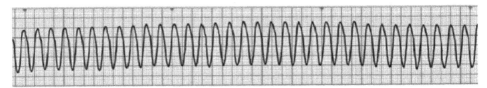

Figure 3.1 Rhythm strip

Reproduced from *Care of the Acutely Ill Adult: An Essential Guide for Nurses*, Creed F and Spiers C, Figure 13.11 © 2010 Oxford University Press. Reproduced with permission of the Licensor through PLSclear

As you arrive, the patient has a cardiac arrest. The rhythm strip is shown in Figure 3.1.

a) What does the rhythm strip show? *(1 mark)*

b) Outline how you would proceed *(10 marks)*

During the second cycle of CPR the nurse asks the following questions:

c) 'What's the most likely cause of the cardiac arrest?' *(1 mark)*

d) 'What is the cause of the local anaesthetic toxicity?' *(1 mark)*

e) 'I've disconnected the epidural. Is there anything else we should do if this arrest was caused by local anaesthetic toxicity?' *(2 marks)*

f) 'What's the dose of intravenous lipid emulsion?' *(5 marks)*

Answers

a) What does the rhythm strip show? *(1 mark)*
  - Ventricular tachycardia

b) Outline how you would proceed *(10 marks)*
  - Confirm cardiorespiratory arrest
  - Call for help
  - Start chest compressions and ventilation at a ratio of 30:2
  - Attach the defibrillator and deliver a shock at 150 J
  - Consider a further two immediate shocks at 150 J (monitored pulseless cardiac arrest with a shockable rhythm)
  - Start 2-minute cycles of minimally interrupted CPR
  - Consider reversible causes
  - Disconnect the epidural infusion
  - Give 1 mg of intravenous adrenaline after the third shock and every 3–5 minutes
  - Give 300 mg of intravenous amiodarone after the third shock

c) 'What's the most likely cause of the cardiac arrest?' *(1 mark)*
  - Local anaesthetic systemic toxicity

d) 'What is the cause of the local anaesthetic toxicity?' *(1 mark)*
  - Intravascular epidural catheter

e) 'I've disconnected the epidural. Is there anything else we should do if this arrest was caused by local anaesthetic toxicity?' *(2 marks)*
  - Administer intravenous lipid emulsion
  - Hyperventilation

f) 'What's the dose of intravenous lipid emulsion?' *(5 marks)*
  - Initial 1.5 mL/kg bolus
  - Further boluses of 1.5 mL/kg at 5 min intervals if the patient remains in cardiac arrest (maximum 3)
  - Infusion of 15 mL/kg/hour
  - Double the infusion rate after 5 minutes if the patient remains in cardiac arrest
  - Maximum cumulative dose of 12 mL/kg

Notes

While needing to insert an epidural catheter is rare for intensive care clinicians, it is common to care for patients with epidurals postoperatively.

Further reading

Association of Anaesthetists of Great Britain and Ireland (AAGBI). Safety guideline: management of severe local anaesthetic toxicity. 2010. Available at: https://www.aagbi.org/sites/default/files/la_toxicity_2010_0.pdf [accessed 9 September 2018].

Christie LE, Pickard J, Weinberg GL. Local anaesthetic systemic toxicity. *BJA Education* 2015;15:136–142.

FFICM syllabus references 1.1, 1.2, 2.2, 2.3, 3.10, 4.1, 5.16, 11.6, 12.7.
CoBaTrICE domains 1, 2, 3, 4, 5, 6.

OSCE 3 station 3—data

Questions

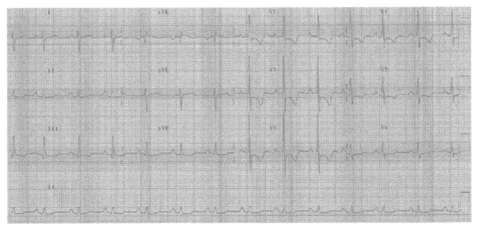

Figure 3.2 Electrocardiogram (ECG)

Reproduced from *Emergencies in Cardiology, Second Edition*, Myerson SG et al., Figure 13.3. © 2009 Oxford University Press. Reproduced with permission of the Licensor through PLSclear

A patient presents with type 2 respiratory failure. The chest X-ray shows hyperexpanded lungs but no consolidation.

An echocardiogram shows normal right and left ventricular contractility. The patient's electrocardiogram (ECG) is shown in Figure 3.2.

a) Describe the ECG *(5 marks)*

b) What ECG findings are typical of right ventricular hypertrophy? *(3 marks)*

c) What is the most likely underlying diagnosis causing the respiratory failure? *(1 mark)*

d) What syndrome describes hypoxaemic respiratory disease and associated structural changes in the right ventricle? *(1 mark)*

The patient is noted to have swollen ankles.

e) What is the cause of peripheral oedema in cor pulmonale with preserved ventricular function? *(1 mark)*

f) What echocardiogram findings help to differentiate between acute and chronic cor pulmonale? *(3 marks)*

g) What are the long-term benefits of oxygen therapy in the management of chronic cor pulmonale? *(1 mark)*

h) What are the effects of mechanical ventilation on the right ventricle? *(2 marks)*

i) Why are pulmonary vasodilators used with caution in patients with cor pulmonale secondary to chronic obstructive pulmonary disease? *(1 mark)*

j) What is the value of N-terminal pro-brain natriuretic peptide (NT pro-BNP) testing for the diagnosis of heart failure in critical care? *(2 marks)*

Answers

a) Describe the ECG *(5 marks)*
- Sinus rhythm
- Prominent P waves (P pulmonale)
- Right axis deviation
- Prominent R waves in V1–3
- T-wave inversion in V1–5, aVF, and III

b) What ECG findings are typical of right ventricular hypertrophy? *(3 marks)*

(1 mark per feature to a maximum of 3)
- Right axis deviation
- Prominent R wave in V1
- T-wave inversion in the precordial leads, most prominent in V1 and inferiorly
- Dominant S wave in V5 or V6

c) What is the most likely underlying diagnosis causing the respiratory failure? *(1 mark)*
- Exacerbation of chronic obstructive pulmonary disease

d) What syndrome describes hypoxaemic respiratory disease and associated structural changes in the right ventricle? *(1 mark)*
- Cor pulmonale

e) What is the cause of peripheral oedema in cor pulmonale with preserved ventricular function? *(1 mark)*
- Chronic hypoxia causes sympathetic stimulation. This results in renin release and subsequent retention of fluid

f) What echocardiogram findings help to differentiate between acute and chronic cor pulmonale? *(3 marks)*
- Significant right ventricular hypertrophy is a feature of chronic cor pulmonale
- The hypertrophied ventricle of chronic cor pulmonale is able to generate higher systolic pressures (>35 mmHg) and high pressure jets of tricuspid regurgitation (>60 mmHg). Such pressures are not seen in acute cor pulmonale
- A dilated right ventricle signifies either acute cor pulmonale or late chronic cor pulmonale (i.e. a non-dilated right ventricle is a feature of the earlier stages of chronic cor pulmonale)

g) What are the long-term benefits of oxygen therapy in the management of chronic cor pulmonale? *(1 mark)*
- To prevent progression to failure of the right ventricle, thereby prolonging life expectancy and improving healthcare-related quality of life

h) What are the effects of mechanical ventilation on the right ventricle? *(2 marks)*
- The increase in intrathoracic pressure reduces venous return (preload) ...
- ... and increases right ventricular afterload

i) Why are pulmonary vasodilators used with caution in patients with cor pulmonale secondary to chronic obstructive pulmonary disease? *(1 mark)*
- Reversal of hypoxic pulmonary vasoconstriction may worsen hypoxaemia

j) What is the value of NT pro-BNP testing for the diagnosis of heart failure in critical care? *(2 marks)*
- A normal NT pro-BNP in the untreated patient has a high negative predictive value, so is useful for ruling out heart failure
- NT pro-BNP has a low specificity in the critical care population therefore a high level is not diagnostic for heart failure

Further reading

Condliffe R, Kiely DG. Critical care management of pulmonary hypertension. *BJA Education* 2017;7:228–234.
Shujaat A, Minkin R, Eden E. Pulmonary hypertension and chronic cor pulmonale in COPD. *International Journal of COPD* 2007;2:273–282.

FFICM syllabus references 1.1, 2.3, 2.6, 3.1, 3.2, 3.3.
CoBaTrICE domains 1, 2, 3.

OSCE 3 station 4—data

Questions

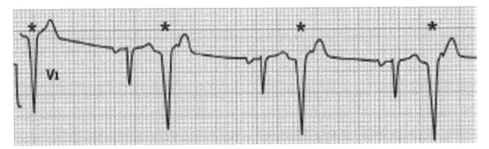

Figure 3.3 Rhythm strip

Reproduced from *Oxford Handbook of Clinical Medicine, Tenth Edition*, Wilkinson IB, Raine T, and Wiles K, Figure 3.34. © 2017 Oxford University Press. Reproduced with permission of the Licensor through PLSclear

Look at the rhythm strip shown in Figure 3.3.

a) How would you describe the complexes marked with a star and what is the rhythm? *(2 marks)*

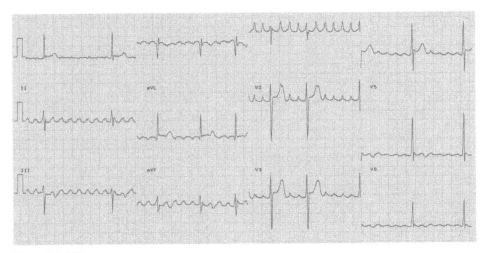

Figure 3.4 ECG

Reproduced from *Emergencies in Cardiology, Second Edition*, Myerson SG *et al.*, Figure 21.31. © 2009 Oxford University Press. Reproduced with permission of the Licensor through PLSclear

Look at Figure 3.4.

b) What abnormalities are shown on this ECG and what is the rhythm? *(6 marks)*

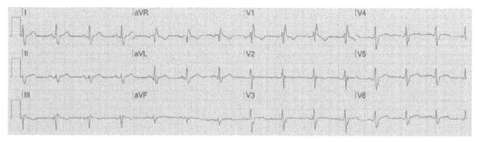

Figure 3.5 ECG

Look at Figure 3.5.

c) What abnormalities are shown on this ECG and what is the rhythm? *(3 marks)*

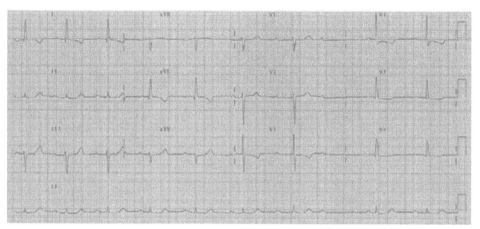

Figure 3.6 ECG

Look at Figure 3.6.

d) What abnormalities are shown on this ECG and what is the rhythm? *(5 marks)*

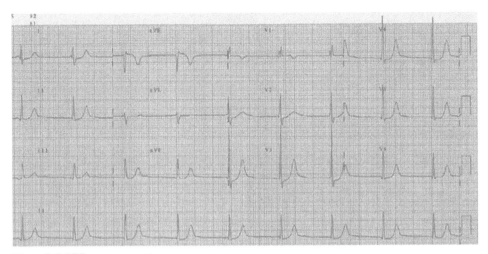

Figure 3.7 ECG

Reproduced from Emergencies in Cardiology, *Second Edition*, Myerson SG et al., Figure 21.24. © 2009 Oxford University Press. Reproduced with permission of the Licensor through PLSclear

Look at Figure 3.7.

e) What abnormalities are shown on this ECG and what is the rhythm? *(4 marks)*

Answers

a) How would you describe the complexes marked with a star and what is the rhythm? *(2 marks)*
  - Premature ventricular contractions or ventricular ectopic beats
  - Ventricular bigeminy
b) What abnormalities are shown on this ECG and what is the rhythm? *(6 marks)*
  - Atrial tachycardia
  - Large bifid P waves
  - Irregular ventricular contractions
  - Ventricular bradycardia
  - ST elevation in I, aVL, and V2–4
  - Atrial flutter with variable conduction
c) What abnormalities are shown on this ECG and what is the rhythm? *(3 marks)*
  - Right bundle branch block
  - Left axis deviation
  - Bifascicular block
d) What abnormalities are shown on this ECG and what is the rhythm? *(5 marks)*
  - Bradycardia
  - T-wave inversion I, aVL, V3–6
  - Progressive PR widening
  - Dropped QRS complex
  - Mobitz type 1 (Wenckebach) second-degree atrioventricular block
e) What abnormalities are shown on this ECG and what is the rhythm? *(4 marks)*

  - Bradycardia
  - Absent P waves
  - Dominant R wave in V1
  - Junctional bradycardia

Notes

There are numerous ECG libraries either online or published but a relatively small number of common rhythm disturbances. It's worth looking at as many sources as possible until you're confident you could identify them in an exam situation.

FFICM syllabus references 2.3, 3.10, 5.11.
CoBaTrICE domain 2.

OSCE 3 station 5—data

Questions

A patient with severe acute respiratory distress syndrome has a PaO_2 of 5.3 kPa (40 mmHg) despite being invasively ventilated using the following ventilator settings:

- Mode—constant pressure, variable flow, mandatory ventilation
- Inspiratory pressure—30 cmH_2O (22 mmHg)
- Expiratory pressure (positive end-expiratory pressure)—14 cmH_2O (10 mmHg)
- Inspiratory:expiratory ratio—1:1
- Rate—22 breaths per minute

a) How is the oxygenation index (OI) calculated, and what would the OI be for this patient? *(2 marks)*

The patient is referred for treatment with extracorporeal membrane oxygenation (ECMO).

b) Which cannulation configurations are used for ECMO therapy? *(3 marks)*
c) What are the disadvantages of venoarterial (VA) compared to venovenous (VV) ECMO? *(3 marks)*
d) What are the potential cannulation options for VV ECMO? *(2 marks)*
e) How might VV ECMO improve a patient's haemodynamic status? *(2 marks)*

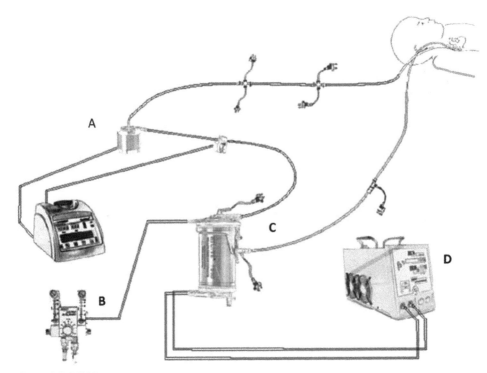

Figure 3.8 ECMO circuit

Reproduced from *Oxford Textbook of Critical Care, Second Edition*, Webb A, et al., Figure 104.4. © 2016 Oxford University Press. Reproduced with permission of the Licensor through PLSclear

Look at Figure 3.8.

f) Identify the components labelled A–D *(4 marks)*

After commencing ECMO the patient's arterial saturations remain low (83%). Access pressures are satisfactory, and the oxygenator and blender are functioning well.

g) What should be done to improve the patient's oxygenation? *(1 mark)*

The patient's saturations remain unchanged after an increase in blood flow.

h) What is the most likely explanation for this? *(1 mark)*

i) What options are available to reduce recirculation of oxygenated blood in the ECMO circuit? *(2 marks)*

Answers

a) How is the oxygenation index (OI) calculated and what would the OI be for this patient?
(2 marks)
- OI = (FiO$_2$ × 100 × mean airway pressure)/PaO$_2$ (mean airway pressure and PaO$_2$ must be in the same unit of measurement)
- (1.0 × 100 × 16)/40 = 1600/40 = 40

b) Which cannulation configurations are used for ECMO therapy? *(3 marks)*
- Venovenous
- Central cannulation
- Venoarterial

c) What are the disadvantages of venoarterial (VA) compared to venovenous (VV) ECMO?
(3 marks)

(1 mark per disadvantage to a maximum of 3)
- Risks of arterial cannulation—injury, dissection, pseudoaneurysm, bleeding
- Risk of arterial embolization
- Potential for impaired pulmonary, coronary, and cerebral perfusion
- Increased left ventricular afterload

d) What are the potential cannulation options for VV ECMO? *(2 marks)*

(1 mark per option to a maximum of 2)
- Internal jugular vein and femoral vein
- Bifemoral venous cannulation
- Single (dual-lumen) cannula

e) How might VV ECMO improve a patient's haemodynamic status? *(2 marks)*
- Improved venous return
- Improved right ventricular function by enabling rest ventilation (lowering right ventricular afterload)

f) Identify the components labelled A–D *(4 marks)*
- A—centrifugal pump
- B—blender
- C—oxygenator
- D—heat exchanger

g) What should be done to improve the patient's oxygenation? *(1 mark)*
- Increase the blood flow rate (pump speed)

h) What is the most likely explanation for this? *(1 mark)*
- Recirculation of oxygenated blood within the ECMO circuit

i) What options are available to reduce recirculation of oxygenated blood in the ECMO circuit?
(2 marks)

(1 mark per option to a maximum of 2)
- Adjust cannula position
- Use a dual-lumen single cannula
- Change to VA ECMO

Notes

Most candidates (and examiners) will have no practical experience of ECMO other than perhaps making a referral. That unfortunately does not mean that it could not appear in the exam.

Further reading

Pavlushkov E, Berman M, Valchanov K. Cannulation techniques for extracorporeal life support. *Annals of Translational Medicine* 2017;5:70.

FFICM syllabus references 3.8, 4.6, 5.1.
CoBaTrICE domain 4.

OSCE 3 station 6—data

Questions

A 4-year-old child is brought to the emergency department by his parents. He has a widespread non-blanching purpuric rash and is cold and listless.

a) What is the most likely diagnosis? *(1 mark)*
b) How would you estimate the weight for this child and what would it be? *(2 marks)*
c) What would be the initial fluid bolus volume for a 16 kg child with septic shock? *(1 mark)*
d) What is the significance of a fluid requirement of 60 mL/kg or more in paediatric sepsis? *(2 marks)*
e) By what formula is the endotracheal tube size (uncuffed) determined, and what size should be used for this child? *(2 marks)*
f) What are the advantages of using a cuffed tube and how does sizing differ from an uncuffed tube? *(4 marks)*
g) A Gram-positive diplococcus is grown from initial blood cultures. What is the likely pathogen? *(1 mark)*
h) Which intracranial complications can result from pneumococcal septicaemia? *(5 marks)*
i) What is the role of early administration of dexamethasone in children with bacterial meningitis? *(2 marks)*

Answers

a) What is the most likely diagnosis? *(1 mark)*
- Meningococcal septicaemia

b) How would you estimate the weight for this child and what would it be? *(2 marks)*
- (Age + 4) × 2 or (age × 2) + 8
- 16 kg

c) What would be the initial fluid bolus volume for a 16 kg child with septic shock? *(1 mark)*
- 320 mL (20 mL/kg)

d) What is the significance of a fluid requirement of 60 mL/kg or more in paediatric sepsis? *(2 marks)*
- There is a high likelihood of developing pulmonary oedema ...
- ... so preparation for intubation is recommended

e) By what formula is the endotracheal tube size (uncuffed) determined and what size should be used for this child? *(2 marks)*
- Age/4 + 4
- Size 5 mm endotracheal tube

f) What would be the advantages of a cuffed tube and how does sizing differ from an uncuffed tube? *(4 marks)*
- Reduced likelihood of tube exchange
- Reduced leak
- Improved performance if higher ventilation pressures are required
- Typically, a half to one size smaller internal diameter tube is used

g) A Gram-positive diplococcus is grown from initial blood cultures. What is the likely pathogen? *(1 mark)*
- *Streptococcus pneumoniae*

h) Which intracranial complications can result from pneumococcal septicaemia? *(5 marks)*

   (1 mark per complication to a maximum of 5)
- Meningitis
- Cerebral abscess
- Subdural empyema
- Cerebral infarction
- Cerebral oedema
- Cranial nerve palsy

i) What is the role of early administration of dexamethasone in children with bacterial meningitis? *(2 marks)*
- Dexamethasone reduces the incidence of hearing loss and neurological sequelae ...
- ... but does not reduce overall mortality

Further reading

Kawasaki T. Update on pediatric sepsis: a review. *Journal of Intensive Care* 2017;5:47.

FFICM syllabus references 2.4, 9.1.
CoBaTrICE domain 9.

OSCE 3 station 7—data

Questions

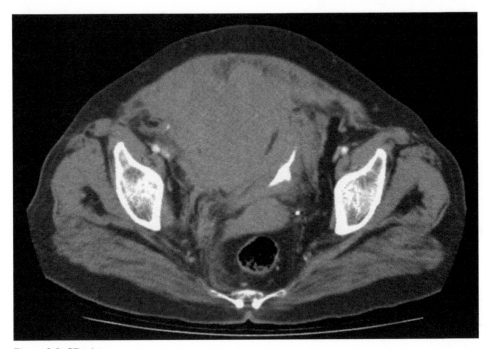

Figure 3.9 CT pelvis

A 70-year-old man taking rivaroxaban for atrial fibrillation has developed back pain and hypotension 2 hours post coronary angiography via the femoral artery. A computed tomography (CT) scan has been performed and is shown in Figure 3.9.

a) What abnormal finding is shown on this CT image? *(1 mark)*

b) What are the common causes of retroperitoneal haemorrhage? *(5 marks)*

c) What is Grey Turner's sign and how long does it typically take to appear? *(2 marks)*

d) List three major complications of a retroperitoneal haematoma *(4 marks)*

e) What management approach should be taken after development of a retroperitoneal haematoma? *(4 marks)*

f) How can coagulopathy due to direct oral anticoagulants (DOACs) be managed? *(4 marks)*

Answers

a) What abnormal finding is shown on this CT image? *(1 mark)*
- Retroperitoneal haematoma

b) What are the common causes of retroperitoneal haemorrhage? *(5 marks)*
- Trauma
- Ruptured abdominal aortic aneurysm
- Interventional vascular procedures, e.g. after femoral artery cannulation
- Haemorrhagic pancreatitis
- Spontaneous—usually in the presence of anticoagulation or antiplatelets

c) What is Grey Turner's sign and how long does it typically take to appear? *(2 marks)*
- Bruising of the flank seen following retroperitoneal bleeding
- 24–48 hours

d) List three major complications of a retroperitoneal haematoma *(4 marks)*

(1 mark per complication to a maximum of 4)
- Abdominal compartment syndrome
- Femoral neuropathy
- Renal impairment
- Infection
- Hypovolaemia (and other complications of haemorrhage)

e) What management approach should be taken after development of a retroperitoneal haematoma? *(4 marks)*
- Volume resuscitation including blood administration and correction of coagulopathy
- Haemorrhage control (surgical, endovascular, or embolization) in the unstable patient
- Conservative management may be considered for haemodynamically stable patients to prevent further bleeding or the introduction of infection
- A period of in-patient observation for major complications

f) How can coagulopathy due to direct oral anticoagulants (DOACs) be managed? *(4 marks)*
- Idarucizumab as a reversal agent for dabigatran
- Non-specific agents including prothrombin concentrates, activated prothrombin concentrates, and recombinant factor VIIa are sometimes recommended
- Tranexamic acid is recommended in most guidelines for life-threatening bleeding although it has no effect on the DOAC pathway
- Haemodialysis or filtration can be effective in removing dabigatran

Further reading

Raval AN, Cigarroa JE, Chung MK, Diaz-Sandoval LJ, Diercks D, Piccini JP, et al. Management of patients on non-vitamin K antagonist oral anticoagulants in the acute care and periprocedural setting: a scientific statement from the American Heart Association. *Circulation* 2017;135:e604–e633.

FFICM syllabus references 1.5, 2.6, 3.1.
CoBaTrICE domains 1, 2.

OSCE 3 station 8—data

Questions

You have been asked to review a 28-year-old woman in the emergency department with an acute exacerbation of asthma.

a) Which clinical signs characterize acute asthma as being life-threatening? *(7 marks)*

b) A peak expiratory flow rate below which value would define asthma as being life-threatening *(1 mark)*

c) What medications should be given as initial treatment of acute life-threatening asthma? *(4 marks)*

d) What medications should be considered if there is a poor response to initial therapy? *(2 marks)*

The patient exhibited signs of life-threatening asthma and was admitted to the critical care unit where she required invasive ventilation with deep sedation. Muscle relaxation was also required due to patient–ventilator dyssynchrony.

Tidal volumes remained low (<150 mL) with the following ventilator settings:

- Inspiratory pressure: 30 cmH$_2$O
- Positive end-expiratory pressure (PEEP): 5 cmH$_2$O
- Rate: 20 breaths per minute

The patient also required an intravenous fluid bolus and an adrenaline infusion because of hypotension. There were no clinical or radiological signs of pneumothorax.

e) What is the most likely explanation for this clinical picture? *(1 mark)*

f) What ventilatory strategies can be employed to manage dynamic hyperinflation? *(5 marks)*

Answers

a) Which clinical signs characterize acute asthma as being life-threatening? *(7 marks)*
- Altered conscious level
- Exhaustion
- Arrhythmias
- Hypotension
- Cyanosis
- Silent chest
- Poor respiratory effort

b) A peak expiratory flow rate below which value would define asthma as being life-threatening *(1 mark)*
- <33% best or predicted

c) What medications should be given as initial treatment of acute life-threatening asthma? *(4 marks)*
- Supplementary oxygen with target saturations of 94–98%
- Beta-2 agonist (nebulized or intravenous)
- Ipratropium bromide (nebulized)
- Steroids (oral or intravenous)

d) What medications should be considered if there is a poor response to initial therapy? *(2 marks)*
- Magnesium sulphate (intravenous)
- Aminophylline (intravenous)

e) What is the most likely explanation for this clinical picture? *(1 mark)*
- Dynamic hyperinflation

f) What ventilatory strategies can be employed to manage dynamic hyperinflation? *(5 marks)*
- Reduction of the tidal volume
- Shortening of the inspiratory time by increasing the inspiratory flow rate, resulting in an increased inspiratory:expiratory ratio
- Reduction of the respiratory rate
- Reduction/removal of extrinsic PEEP
- Intermittent disconnection and manual chest decompression

Further reading

British Thoracic Society/Scottish Intercollegiate Guidelines Network (SIGN). *British Guideline on the Management of Asthma: A National Clinical Guideline*. SIGN Report Number 153. 2016. Edinburgh: SIGN.

FFICM syllabus references 1.7, 2.5, 2.7, 3.1, 4.6, 5.2.
CoBaTrICE domains 1, 2, 3, 4, 5.

OSCE 3 station 9—data

Questions

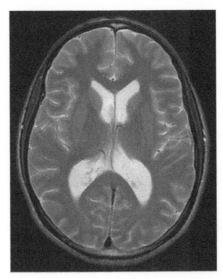

Figure 3.10 MRI brain
Reproduced from *Oxford Textbook of Medicine, Fifth Edition*, Warrell D, et al., Figure 24.3.3.1b. © 2010 Oxford University Press.
Reproduced with permission of the Licensor through PLSclear

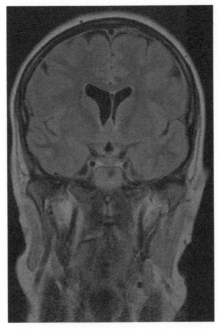

Figure 3.11 MRI brain
Reproduced from *Oxford Textbook of Medicine, Fifth Edition*, Warrell D, et al., Figure 24.3.3.1d. © 2010 Oxford University Press.
Reproduced with permission of the Licensor through PLSclear

Look at Figures 3.10 and 3.11.

a) Describe the anatomical plane and magnetic resonance imaging (MRI) sequence for each of the images *(4 marks)*

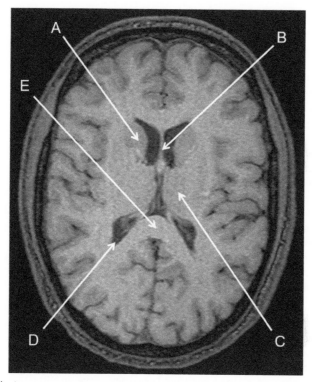

Figure 3.12 MRI brain

Reproduced from *Oxford Textbook of Medicine, Fifth Edition*, Warrell D, et al., Figure 24.3.3.1c. © 2010 Oxford University Press. Reproduced with permission of the Licensor through PLSclear

Look at Figure 3.12.

b) What are the structures labelled A–E? *(5 marks)*

c) How is an MRI image generated? *(3 marks)*

d) What are the absolute contraindications to MRI? *(3 marks)*

e) What monitoring issues need to be considered when performing an MRI scan in a patient requiring mechanical ventilation? *(5 marks)*

Answers

a) Describe the anatomical plane and magnetic resonance imaging (MRI) sequence for each of the images *(4 marks)*
  - Figure 3.11:
    - Axial
    - T2 weighted
  - Figure 3.12:
    - Coronal
    - Fluid-attenuated inversion recovery (FLAIR)
b) What are the structures labelled A–E? *(5 marks)*
  - A—caudate nucleus
  - B—septum pellucidum
  - C—thalamus
  - D—occipital horn of the lateral ventricle
  - E—corpus callosum
c) How is an MRI image generated? *(3 marks)*
  - A powerful magnet is applied to align the usually randomly aligned protons in tissue water
  - The protons are then displaced from their alignment by application of a radiofrequency pulse. When this radiofrequency pulse terminates, the protons realign themselves with the main magnetic field
  - This realignment releases several radiofrequency signals, which are detected, processed, and turned into an image
d) What are the absolute contraindications to MRI? *(3 marks)*

  (1 mark per contraindication to a maximum of 3)
  - Cochlear implants
  - Pacemakers, implantable cardiac defibrillators, and some metallic heart valves
  - Metallic intraocular foreign bodies
  - Ferromagnetic clips (especially neurosurgical)
e) What monitoring issues need to be considered when performing an MRI scan in a patient requiring mechanical ventilation? *(5 marks)*
  - All equipment needs to be MRI compatible (non-ferromagnetic) including use of fibre-optic or carbon fibre cabling
  - All MRI incompatible monitoring should be placed in the control room outside of the magnet environment
  - Visual alarms should be used because of the noise from the MRI scanner
  - Braided, short, MRI-compatible electrocardiogram leads should be placed in a narrow triangle on the chest to prevent interference
  - Because of the required length of tubing, there may be a delay when using MRI-incompatible end-tidal carbon dioxide monitoring

Notes

MRI image sequences probably fall into the category of 'just memorize it for the exam' unless you work in neurointensive care.

Further reading

Molyneux AJ, Renowden S, Bradley M. Imaging in neurological diseases. Warrell DA, Cox TM, Firth JD (eds.) *Oxford Textbook of Medicine*, 5th Edition, pp. 4768–4781. Oxford: Oxford University Press; 2010.

FFICM syllabus references 2.6, 10.1.
CoBaTrICE domains 2, 10.

OSCE 3 station 10—data

Questions

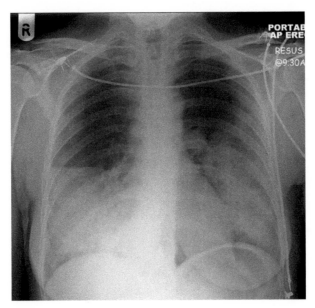

Figure 3.13 Chest X-ray
Reproduced from *Advanced Respiratory Critical Care*, Hughes M and Black R, Figure 6.10. © 2011 Oxford University Press.
Reproduced with permission of the Licensor through PLSclear

A 45-year-old woman has presented to the emergency department with a 3-day history of fever, rigors, and a cough productive of green sputum. Her oxygen saturation is 86% on air and 91% on high-flow oxygen. Her respiratory rate is 38 breaths per minute and her temperature is 38.4°C. She has no significant past medical history and has not had any recent hospital admissions.

Look at Figure 3.13.

a) What is the diagnosis? *(1 mark)*
b) Which lobes are affected by the pneumonia? *(2 marks)*
c) What is the purpose of the CURB-65 score? *(2 marks)*
d) What parameters including values make up the CURB-65 score? *(5 marks)*
e) What are the organisms which most commonly cause community-acquired pneumonia (CAP) necessitating critical care admission in Europe? *(3 marks)*

The patient is noted to have a pleural effusion.

f) What are the three different types of para-pneumonic effusions? *(3 marks)*

The legionella urinary antigen test is positive.

g) What are the potential non-respiratory complications of infection with *Legionella* spp.? *(4 marks)*

Answers

a) What is the diagnosis? *(1 mark)*
  - Bilateral community-acquired pneumonia
b) Which lobes are affected by the pneumonia? *(2 marks)*
  - Right middle lobe
  - Left lower lobe
c) What is the purpose of the CURB-65 score? *(2 marks)*
  - To assess severity ...
  - ... and to predict mortality in CAP
d) What parameters including values make up the CURB-65 score? *(5 marks)*
  - C—Confusion: new-onset confusion (mini mental test ≤8)
  - U—Urea: >7 mmol/L
  - R—Respiratory rate: ≥30 breaths per minute
  - B—Blood pressure (BP): systolic BP <90 mmHg or diastolic BP ≤60 mmHg
  - 65—Age: ≥65 years
  (Reproduced from *Thorax*, Lim WS et al., Defining community acquired pneumonia severity on presentation to hospital: an international derivation and validation study, 58, 5, pp. 377–382, Copyright 2003, with permission from BMJ Publishing Group Ltd.)

e) What are the organisms which most commonly cause CAP necessitating critical care admission in Europe? *(3 marks)*

  (1 mark per organism to a maximum of 3)
  - *Streptococcus pneumonia*
  - *Legionella pneumophila*
  - *Staphylococcus aureus*
  - *Haemophilus influenza*
  - *Pseudomonas aeruginosa*
f) What are the three different types of para-pneumonic effusions? *(3 marks)*
  - Uncomplicated—sterile pleural fluid
  - Complicated—bacterial invasion without pus, a clear fluid with pH <7.2
  - Empyema—pus in the pleural space
g) What are the potential non-respiratory complications of infection with *Legionella* spp.? *(4 marks)*

  (1 mark per complication up to a maximum of 4 marks)
  - Encephalitis
  - Pericarditis
  - Pancreatitis
  - Polyarthropathy
  - Hyponatraemia
  - Abnormal liver function
  - Thrombocytopenia
  - Diarrhoea
  - Renal function

Further reading

Bakere H, Halpin D. Treatment of specific diseases: pneumonia. In: Hughes M, Grant I, Black R (eds.) *Advanced Respiratory Critical Care*, pp. 493–514. Oxford: Oxford University Press; 2011.

FFICM syllabus references 1.1, 2.6, 3.1, 3.9, 11.7.
CoBaTrICE domain 2.

OSCE 3 station 11—data

Questions

You are asked to review a 69-year-old woman in the emergency department with respiratory distress. She is a lifelong smoker and known to have chronic obstructive pulmonary disease (COPD). Her arterial blood gas (ABG) test results on 4 L of oxygen are (normal ranges in brackets):

- pH 7.28 (7.35–7.45)
- PCO_2 7.9 kPa (4.7–6.0 kPa)
- PO_2 9.3 kPa (>10.6 kPa)
- HCO_3^- 34 mmol/L (24–30 mmol/L)
- Base excess +4 mmol/L (+/− 2 mmol/L)

a) What do these ABG results show? *(2 marks)*
b) What are the indications for non-invasive ventilation (NIV) in acute exacerbations of COPD (AECOPD)? *(3 marks)*
c) What is the first-choice interface for delivering NIV? *(1 mark)*
d) What are the absolute contraindications to fixed face mask NIV in AECOPD? *(4 marks)*
e) What should be the target oxygen saturations for a patient with AECOPD receiving NIV? *(1 mark)*
f) What are the potential complications of NIV? *(4 marks)*
g) What are the indications for invasive mechanical ventilation in patients with AECOPD? *(5 marks)*

Answers

a) What do these ABG results show? *(2 marks)*
- Partially compensated respiratory acidosis
- Hypoxaemia

b) What are the indications for non-invasive ventilation (NIV) in acute exacerbations of COPD (AECOPD)? *(3 marks)*
- A pH <7.35 ...
- ... and pCO_2 >6.5 kPa ...
- ... persisting after optimal medical therapy

c) What is the first-choice interface for delivering NIV? *(1 mark)*
- Full face mask

d) What are the absolute contraindications to full face mask NIV in AECOPD? *(4 marks)*
- Patient refusal
- Severe facial deformity
- Facial burns
- Fixed upper airway obstruction

e) What should be the target oxygen saturations for a patient with AECOPD receiving NIV? *(1 mark)*
- 88–92%

f) What are the potential complications of NIV? *(4 marks)*

(1 mark per complication to a maximum of 4)
- Nasal bridge ulceration or skin irritation
- Nasal mucosal drying/ulceration
- Gastric distension
- Sinus/ear canal discomfort
- Anxiety/agitation
- Pneumothorax
- Hypotension
- Raised intracranial/intraocular pressure

g) What are the indications for invasive mechanical ventilation in patients with AECOPD? *(5 marks)*
- Imminent respiratory arrest
- Severe respiratory distress/exhaustion
- Contraindications to NIV
- Persisting pH <7.15 or deterioration in pH despite NIV
- Coma or worsening level of consciousness despite NIV

Further reading

Davidson AC, Banham S, Elliott M, Kennedy D, Gelder C, Glossop A, et al. BTS/ICS guideline for the ventilatory management of acute hypercapnic respiratory failure in adults. *Thorax* 2016;71 Suppl 2:ii1–35.

FFICM syllabus references 1.1, 2.5, 3.1, 3.8, 4.6.
CoBaTrICE domains 1, 2, 3, 4.

OSCE 3 station 12—equipment

Questions

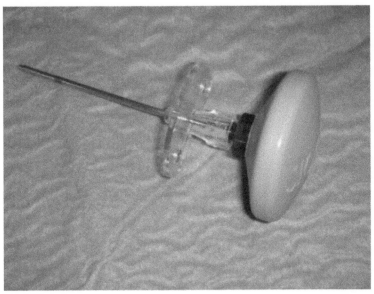

Figure 3.14 Medical device

Reproduced from *A Resuscitation Room Guide*, Banerjee A and Hargreaves C, Figure 6.3. © 2007 Oxford University Press. Reproduced with permission of the Licensor through PLSclear

Look at Figure 3.14.

a) What is this device? *(1 mark)*
b) What are the contraindications to intraosseous (IO) needle insertion? *(3 marks)*
c) What sites are commonly used for IO access? *(3 marks)*
d) How can the position of an IO needle be confirmed clinically? *(4 marks)*
e) What are the complications of IO insertion and use? *(3 marks)*
f) When taking blood samples from an IO device, which parameters correlate poorly with venous plasma values? *(3 marks)*
g) Complete Table 3.1q to show the venous drainage for each IO insertion site *(3 marks)*

Table 3.1q Interosseous venous drainage

Intraosseous insertion site	Vein
Proximal tibia	
Distal tibia	
Proximal humerus	

Answers

a) What is this device? (*1 mark*)
- Intraosseous needle

b) What are the contraindications to intraosseous (IO) needle insertion? (*3 marks*)

(1 mark per contraindication to a maximum of 3)
- Traumatic bone injury at or proximal to the site of insertion
- Vascular interruption to the limb (acute ischaemia or compartment syndrome)
- Burn at the site of insertion
- Skin or bone infection at the site of insertion
- Severe bone fragility, e.g. osteoporosis, osteogenesis imperfecta

c) What sites are commonly used for IO access? (*3 marks*)

(1 mark per site to a maximum of 3)
- Proximal tibia
- Proximal humerus
- Distal tibia
- Distal femur
- Iliac crest

d) How can the position of an IO needle be confirmed clinically? (*4 marks*)
- Loss of resistance on entering the bone marrow
- Stability of the needle
- Aspiration of bone marrow
- Administration of 2 mL of saline without subcutaneous tissue swelling and 10 mL of saline without significant resistance

e) What are the complications of IO insertion and use? (*3 marks*)

(1 mark per complication to a maximum of 3)
- Malposition or displacement
- Pain
- Extravasation
- Compartment syndrome
- Infection
- Injury to underlying structures
- Disruption of the growth plate

f) When taking blood samples from an IO device, which parameters correlate poorly with venous plasma values? (*3 marks*)

(1 mark per parameter to a maximum of 3)
- White cell count
- Platelets
- Sodium
- Potassium
- Calcium
- Carbon dioxide

g) Complete Table 3.1a to show the venous drainage for each IO insertion site *(3 marks)*

Table 3.1a Interosseous venous drainage

Intraosseous insertion site	Vein
Proximal tibia	*Popliteal vein*
Distal tibia	*Great saphenous vein*
Proximal humerus	*Axillary vein*

Further reading

Bradburn S, Gill S, Doane M. Understanding and establishing intraosseous access. World Federation of Society of Anaesthesiologists. 26 June 2015. Tutorial 317. Available at: https://www.wfsahq.org/resources/anaesthesia-tutorial-of-the-week [accessed 4 June 2018].

Petitpas F, Guenezan J, Vendeuvre T, Scepi M, Oriot D, Momoz O. Use of intra-osseous access in adult: a systematic review. *Critical Care* 2016;20:102.

FFICM syllabus references 1.5, 1.6, 2.2.
CoBaTrICE domain 5.

OSCE 3 station 13—equipment

Questions

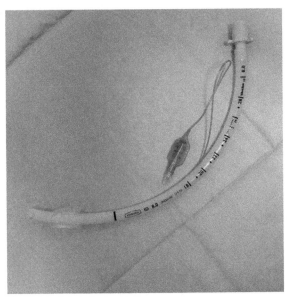

Figure 3.15 Medical device
Reproduced with kind permission from Smiths Medical

Look at Figure 3.15.

a) What is this device? *(1 mark)*
b) What material is an endotracheal tube (ETT) made of? *(1 mark)*
c) What is the Murphy eye and what is its function? *(2 marks)*
d) Why might supraglottic suction be added to an ETT design? *(1 mark)*
e) What is the diameter of the connection at the proximal end of the ETT? *(1 mark)*
f) On a chest X ray, over which vertebral bodies would you expect to see the carina? *(1 mark)*
g) What is the meaning of the code IT or Z79-IT in reference to an ETT *(1 mark)*

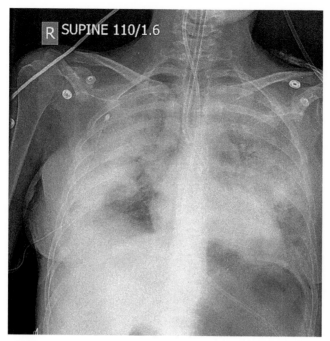

Figure 3.16 Chest X-ray

Look at Figure 3.16.

h) What type of ETT is seen on this chest X-ray? *(1 mark)*
i) What are the possible indications for use of a double-lumen tube (DLT) in critical care? *(3 marks)*
j) How does the bronchial limb of a right-sided DLT differ from that of a left-sided DLT? *(1 mark)*
k) Describe the blind insertion technique for a left-sided DLT *(7 marks)*

Answers

a) What is this device? *(1 mark)*
   • An endotracheal tube

b) What material is an endotracheal tube (ETT) made of? *(1 mark)*
   • Polyvinyl chloride

c) What is the Murphy eye and what is its function? *(2 marks)*
   • A side hole near the tip ...
   • ... to allow gas flow should the end of the tube become occluded

d) Why might supraglottic suction be added to an ETT design? *(1 mark)*
   • To reduce the risk of microaspiration and subsequent ventilator-associated pneumonia

e) What is the diameter of the connection at the proximal end of an ETT? *(1 mark)*
   • 15 mm

f) On a chest X ray, over which vertebral bodies would you expect to see the carina? *(1 mark)*
   • T5–7

g) What is the meaning of the code IT or Z79-IT in reference to an ETT *(1 mark)*
   • The code denotes that the ETT has been tested to confirm tissue compatibility

h) What type of ETT is seen on this chest X-ray? *(1 mark)*
   • Left-sided double-lumen tube

i) What are the possible indications for use of a double-lumen tube (DLT) in critical care? *(3 marks)*

   (1 mark per indication to a maximum of 3)
   • Massive pulmonary haemorrhage
   • Bronchopleural fistula
   • Protection of an undiseased or transplanted lung from pus or high pressures
   • To facilitate whole lung lavage

j) How does the bronchial limb of a right-sided DLT differ from that of a left-sided DLT *(1 mark)*
   • The right-sided tube has a ventilation slot (hole) to allow for the proximal position of the right upper lobe

k) Describe the blind insertion technique for a left-sided DLT *(7 marks)*
   • Insert a stylet into the DLT and perform direct laryngoscopy
   • Insert the DLT through the laryngeal inlet with the curved tip facing anteriorly
   • Remove the stylet, rotate the DLT 90 degrees anticlockwise, and advance until resistance is felt
   • Inflate the tracheal cuff and confirm endotracheal tube placement as usual (end-tidal CO_2, chest auscultation)
   • Open the tracheal cap to air and clamp proximal to the cap. Inflate the bronchial cuff until no leak is felt through the tracheal cap and only the left lung is being ventilated. Release the clamp and replace the cap
   • Open the bronchial cap to air and clamp proximal to the cap. Confirm that only the right lung is being ventilated
   • Confirm position with fibreoptic bronchoscopy

Notes

The first half of this question asks pretty much all there is to know about the endotracheal tube, a device you would be expected to be very familiar with. The second part asks about a device you may not have seen before, let alone used. Our advice would be to see one being inserted if you haven't already; failing that try and get hold of one to play with or look for a reputable video online.

Further reading

Anantham D, Jagadesan R, Tiew PEC. Clinical review: independent lung ventilation in critical care. *Critical Care* 2005;9:594–600.

FFICM syllabus references 2.6, 3.1, 4.6, 5.1, 5.2, 6.4.
CoBaTrICE domain 5.

OSCE 4

OSCE 4 station 1—professionalism

Questions

A patient on the high dependency unit underwent an emergency surgical procedure 2 days ago. Her haemoglobin concentration is 64 g/dL (normal range: 115–160 g/dL) and you decide to prescribe an allogenic blood transfusion pending her consent. She has capacity for decision-making concerning her treatment.

a) What will you tell the patient about the blood transfusion? *(8 marks)*

The patient gives consent for the transfusion.

b) As well as the date and time, what other details of the conversation should be included in the patient record? *(4 marks)*

You are then called to see another patient, who has been intubated and ventilated after sustaining major trauma including life-threatening haemorrhage. During the primary survey they were noted to have 'do not give me a blood transfusion' tattooed on their chest. The resuscitation team all agree that a transfusion is clinically indicated to prevent death.

c) Why does the tattoo not act as a legally binding advanced refusal for blood transfusion? *(4 marks)*

d) What should you do? *(1 mark)*

Answers

a) What will you tell the patient about the blood transfusion? *(8 marks)*

(1 mark per topic to a maximum of 8)
- Explain the rationale and the proposed benefits of the blood transfusion
- Discussion of risks:
  - Incorrect blood administration (1:12,000)
  - Viral infection (HIV 1:6.5 million, hepatitis B 1:1.3 million, hepatitis C 1:28 million, human T-cell lymphotropic virus type 1 (HTLV) 1:18 million)
  - Bacterial infection from contaminated products
  - Allergy including life-threatening anaphylaxis
  - Transfusion-related circulatory overload
  - Transfusion-related acute lung injury
  - Febrile reactions (1:75) and urticaria (1:100)
- Discuss alternatives to transfusion
- Explain that once the patient has been transfused they will no longer be able to give blood
- Ensure understanding and offer time before deciding
- Give the patient an information leaflet

General communication *(3 marks)*
  Marks awarded for behaviours such as the following:
- Eye contact, introduces self, and body language
- Pace and volume of speech
- Demonstrates empathy and addresses concerns
- Offers clear explanations
- Avoids medical jargon

b) As well as the date and time, what other details of the conversation should be included in the patient record? *(4 marks)*
- The information discussed
- The decision that was made
- Any written information that was given to the patient
- Any specific requests made by the patient

c) Why does the tattoo not act as a legally binding advanced refusal for blood transfusion? *(4 marks)*
- The refusal, though written, is not signed or witnessed
- There is no declaration that a blood transfusion should be withheld even if this results in death
- There is no information available about whether the advance refusal was made under free will and that the refusal was an informed decision
- There may also be doubts about the contemporaneous nature of the statement (the tattoo may remain despite the patient changing their mind)

d) What should you do? *(1 mark)*
- Make a best interests decision using the tattoo as non-binding information

Notes

The final two parts of this question are assessing your understanding of advance directives rather than refusal of blood. The same question could, therefore, be asked in different contexts.

Further reading

British Medical Association. Advance decisions and proxy decision-making in medical treatment and research guidance. Available at: bma.org.uk/advice/employment/ethics/mental-capacity [accessed 8 January 2018].

General Medical Council. Consent: patients and doctors making decisions together. 2008. Available at: https://www.gmc-uk.org/guidance [accessed 4 February 2018].

Joint United Kingdom (UK) Blood Transfusion and Tissue Transplantation Services Professional Advisory Committee. Consent for blood transfusion. Available at: https://www.transfusionguidelines.org/transfusion-practice/consent-for-blood-transfusion-1 [accessed 8 January 2018].

FFICM syllabus references 4.3, 11.4, 12.1, 12.3, 12.11, 12.12.
CoBaTrICE domains 11, 12.

OSCE 4 station 2—resuscitation

Questions

You are about to intubate a patient on the critical care unit with worsening hypoxaemia.
   Observations:

- Respiratory rate 35 breaths per minute, SpO$_2$ 92% (FiO$_2$ 0.7 via high-flow nasal cannulae)
- Heart rate 116 beats per minute;, blood pressure 115/60 mmHg
- Glasgow Coma Scale score 14/15

You pre-oxygenate for 3 minutes, then administer the induction and paralysing agents.
   On direct laryngoscopy you cannot see normal anatomical landmarks and are unable to blindly pass the bougie or endotracheal tube.

a) What could you do to improve the view at laryngoscopy? *(6 marks)*

b) What is the recommended maximum number of attempts at laryngoscopy? *(1 mark)*

All attempts to improve the laryngoscopy view and intubate the patient fail.

c) What would you do next? *(4 marks)*

You insert a supraglottic airway device (SAD) but you are unable to ventilate using the device and there is an audible leak.

d) What would your next actions be? *(2 marks)*

e) What type of SAD is recommended by the Difficult Airway Society (DAS)? *(1 mark)*

f) Give an example of a second-generation SAD *(1 mark)*

g) What is the maximum number of attempts at SAD insertion recommended by the DAS? *(1 mark)*

You successfully maintain oxygenation and ventilation using a SAD on your second attempt. The patient is haemodynamically stable.

h) What further options would you consider? *(4 marks)*

Answers

a) What could you do to improve the view at laryngoscopy? *(6 marks)*
   - Optimize head and neck position
   - Ensure adequate neuromuscular blockade
   - Attempt direct laryngoscopy with an alternative design or size of blade
   - Perform video laryngoscopy
   - Request external laryngeal manipulation
   - Remove cricoid pressure

b) What is the recommended maximum number of attempts at laryngoscopy? *(1 mark)*
   - Three plus one attempt by an expert

c) What would you do next? *(4 marks)*
   - Declare a failed intubation
   - Call for help
   - Maintain oxygenation and ventilation using a SAD or a two-person facemask technique with adjuncts
   - Ensure that 'front of neck access' equipment is available

d) What would your next actions be? *(2 marks)*
   - Try a different size and/or type of SAD
   - Open 'front of neck access' equipment

e) What type of SAD is recommended by the Difficult Airway Society (DAS)? *(1 mark)*
   - A second-generation device

f) Give an example of a second-generation SAD *(1 mark)*

   (1 mark per example to a maximum of 1)
   - LMA ProSeal™
   - i-gel™
   - LMA Supreme™
   - SLIPA™

g) What is the maximum number of attempts at SAD insertion recommended by the DAS? *(1 mark)*
   - Three plus one attempt by an expert

h) What further options would you consider? *(4 marks)*
   - Waiting for an expert
   - Waking the patient
   - Intubating the trachea via the SAD
   - Performing a tracheostomy or cricothyroidotomy

Notes

The failed intubation drill is something you should be very familiar with, and it would be very easy for the examiners to ask you to perform it in an OSCE (there are defined actions and the drill doesn't take too long). This is another scenario where you should be efficient but not rush—there will be enough time to complete the scenario and you don't want to miss marks.

Further reading

Difficult Airway Society. ICU intubation guidelines. 2017. Available at: https://www.das.uk.com/guidelines/icu_guidelines2017 [accessed 26 March 2018].

FFICM syllabus references 4.1, 4.6, 5.1, 5.2, 5.3, 11.6, 12.2.
CoBaTrICE domains 4, 5, 11.

OSCE 4 station 3—data

Questions

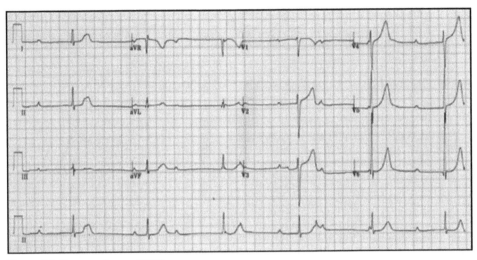

Figure 4.1 Electrocardiogram (ECG)

Reproduced from *Challenging Concepts in Cardiovascular Medicine*, Myat A, Haldar S, and Redwood S, Figure 18.1. © 2011 Oxford University Press. Reproduced with permission of the Licensor through PLSclear

A patient presents to the emergency department complaining of dizziness. They have a blood pressure of 82/49 mmHg.

Look at the electrocardiogram (ECG) in Figure 4.1.

a) What abnormalities are present on this ECG? *(3 marks)*

b) What are the possible routes by which temporary pacing can be delivered? *(3 marks)*

c) Describe how to perform temporary transvenous pacing *(5 marks)*

d) What potential complications are associated with the use of temporary pacing wires? *(2 marks)*

e) Which three clinical signs make up Beck's triad in a patient with acute pericardial tamponade? *(3 marks)*

f) Describe percutaneous drainage of a pericardial tamponade using the subxiphoid landmark technique *(4 marks)*

Answers

a) What abnormalities are present on this ECG? *(3 marks)*

(1 mark per abnormality to a maximum of 3)
- Bradycardia (35 beats per minute)
- Atrioventricular dissociation
- Left ventricular hypertrophy
- Peaked T waves

b) What are the possible routes by which temporary pacing can be delivered? *(3 marks)*

(1 mark per route to a maximum of 3)
- Transcutaneous
- Transvenous
- Epicardial
- Oesophageal

c) Describe how to perform temporary transvenous pacing *(5 marks)*
- Pre-procedure preparation:
  - Consent (often best interests decision due to lack of capacity), monitoring (ECG, blood pressure, pulse oximetry), attach defibrillator pads, intravenous access
- Obtain central venous access:
  - Right internal jugular or subclavian are the preferred sites
- Insert the temporary pacing wire under fluoroscopic or X-ray guidance
- Place the wire in the apex of the right ventricle:
  - Traverse the tricuspid valve (often associated with arrhythmias) and orientate the pacing wire tip to the desired position
- Establish pacing and secure the wire:
  - Connect the temporary pacing wire to the external pacing box—establish pacing threshold, capture threshold, and set pacing programme
  - Secure the wire to the skin and cover with a transparent occlusive dressing
  - Request a post-procedure ECG and chest X-ray

d) What complications are associated with the use of temporary transvenous pacing wires? *(2 marks)*

(1 mark per complication to a maximum of 2)
- During insertion:
  - Introducer insertion—arterial puncture, pneumothorax, air embolus, bleeding
  - Arrhythmias
  - Cardiac perforation and tamponade
- During use:
  - Displacement
  - Venous thrombosis
  - Infection
  - Cardiac perforation and tamponade

e) Which three clinical signs make up Beck's triad in a patient with acute pericardial tamponade? *(3 marks)*
- Low blood pressure
- Distended neck veins
- Quiet, muffled heart sounds

f) Describe percutaneous drainage of a pericardial tamponade using the subxiphoid landmark technique *(4 marks)*
- Obtain consent and establish monitoring for intravenous access
- Position the patient—semi-erect positioning with a slightly left lateral rotation brings the pericardial fluid closer to the chest wall. Create a sterile field
- Prepare the equipment:
  - Pericardiocentesis needle with ECG alligator clip attached to continuous ECG monitoring (precordial lead monitoring is omitted in the blind technique)
  - 50 mL syringe, three-way tap, and collecting tubing and bag for aspiration
- Procedure:
  - Subcutaneous local anaesthetic infiltration between the left costal margin and xiphisternum
  - Blind approach—puncture at the infiltration site, orientate the needle 15–30 degrees to the abdominal wall, and advance the needle (while continuously aspirating) aiming towards the left shoulder. An increase in resistance followed by a pop associated with pain indicates pericardial puncture
  - When using precordial lead monitoring, detection of needle contact with the epicardium is indicated by ST- and PR-segment elevation with ventricular and atrial contact respectively
  - Once correct needle placement is established, withdraw the needle to avoid perforation and aspirate

Notes

This question asks you how to perform two procedures that you are unlikely to have performed, and perhaps have not even seen (but are in the curriculum). Both are essentially performed using the technique as you would imagine it, meaning that if you had come across this question for the first time in the exam it's worth having an educated guess if only to achieve the marks for consent, sterility, intravenous access, etc.

Further reading

De Carlini CC, Maggiolini S. Pericardiocentesis in cardiac tamponade: indications and practical aspects. *E-Journal of Cardiology Practice* 2017;15. Available at: https://www.escardio.org/Journals/E-Journal-of-Cardiology-Practice/Volume-15 [accessed 2 January 2018].

FFICM syllabus references 2.3, 3.1, 4.5, 5.12, 5.13.
CoBaTrICE domains 1, 2, 4, 5.

OSCE 4 station 4—data

Questions

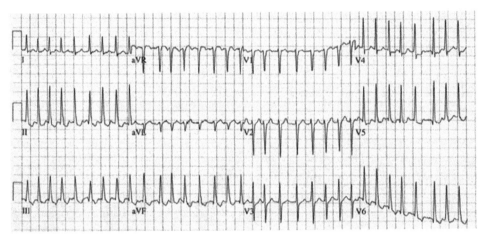

Figure 4.2 Electrocardiogram (ECG)

Reproduced from *Oxford Case Histories in Cardiology*, Rajendram R, Ehtisham J, and Forfar C, Figure 44.1. © 2011 Oxford University Press. Reproduced with permission of the Licensor through PLSclear

A 46-year-old man is admitted to the emergency department after developing palpitations and collapsing during a night out with friends. He tells you that he still feels extremely light headed and took some amphetamine tablets an hour ago. He has a heart rate of 198 beats per minute and blood pressure of 74/52 mmHg. His SpO_2 is 98% on 15 L of oxygen and his respiratory rate is 28 breaths per minute. An electrocardiogram (ECG) is recorded which is shown in Figure 4.2.

a) Describe this ECG *(3 marks)*
b) What treatment is indicated for the atrial fibrillation? *(1 mark)*

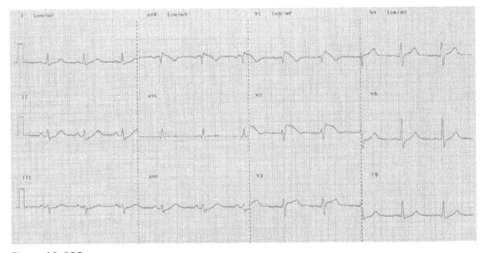

Figure 4.3 ECG

Reproduced from *Emergencies in Cardiology, Second Edition*, Myerson SG et al., Figure 21.39. © 2009 Oxford University Press. Reproduced with permission of the Licensor through PLSclear

A 24-year-old man is admitted to the emergency department complaining of feeling unwell after reportedly taking a large quantity of cocaine. His blood pressure is 240/124 mmHg. An ECG is taken which is shown in Figure 4.3.

c) What abnormalities are present on this ECG? *(2 marks)*

d) What pattern does this ECG demonstrate? *(1 mark)*

e) Which drugs are recommended for the treatment of cocaine-associated hypertension? *(3 marks)*

f) Which group of antihypertensive drugs are to be avoided in cocaine toxicity and why? *(2 marks)*

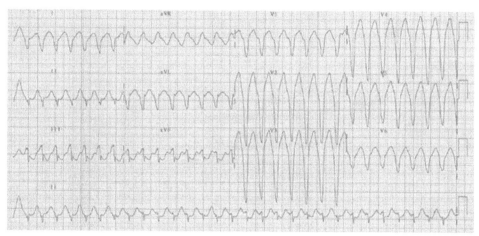

Figure 4.4 ECG

Reproduced from *Emergencies in Cardiology, Second Edition*, Myerson SG et al., Figure 21.35. © 2009 Oxford University Press. Reproduced with permission of the Licensor through PLSclear

There is a change in rhythm on the monitor. The ECG is repeated and is shown in Figure 4.4.

g) What abnormalities are seen on this ECG? *(2 marks)*

h) What intravenous drugs should be considered for treating a haemodynamically stable patient with ventricular tachycardia (VT)? *(4 marks)*

i) Which maintenance therapies should be considered for patients who have had episodes of VT without a treatable cause? *(2 marks)*

Answers

a) Describe this ECG *(3 marks)*
- Atrial fibrillation
- ST-segment depression and T-wave inversion in leads II, III, aVF, and V4–6
- Normal axis and QT interval

b) What treatment is indicated for the atrial fibrillation? *(1 mark)*
- Synchronized DC cardioversion

c) What abnormalities are present on this ECG? *(2 marks)*
- ST elevation in V1–3
- T-wave inversion in V1–2

d) What pattern does this ECG demonstrate? *(1 mark)*
- Drug-induced Brugada

e) Which drugs are recommended for the treatment of cocaine-associated hypertension? *(3 marks)*
- Benzodiazepines (e.g. diazepam)
- Nitrates (e.g. glyceryl trinitrate)
- Phentolamine

f) Which group of antihypertensive drugs are to be avoided in cocaine toxicity and why? *(2 marks)*
- Beta blockers
- Beta blockade can result in unopposed alpha adrenergic stimulation, worsening coronary artery vasoconstriction, and systemic hypertension

g) What abnormalities are seen on this ECG? *(2 marks)*
- Prolonged QRS interval
- Tachycardia

h) What intravenous drugs should be considered for treating a haemodynamically stable patient with VT? *(4 marks)*
- Amiodarone
- Flecainide
- Lignocaine
- Propafenone

i) Which maintenance therapies should be considered for patients who have had episodes of VT without a treatable cause? *(2 marks)*
- Implantable cardiac defibrillator
- Pharmacological prevention with sotalol or amiodarone

Further reading

Johnson NJ, Hollander JE. Management of cocaine poisoning. In: *Oxford Textbook of Critical Care*, 2nd Edition, pp. 1545–1548. Oxford: Oxford University Press; 2016.

National Institute for Health and Care Excellence. Treatment summary—arrhythmias. Available at: https://bnf.nice.org.uk/treatment-summary/arrhythmias.html [accessed 3 November 2018].

FFICM syllabus references 1.1, 1.2, 2.3, 3.1, 3.3, 3.10, 4.1, 5.11.
CoBaTrICE domains 1, 2, 3.

OSCE 4 station 5—data

Questions

A patient presents to hospital with breathlessness. Their pulmonary function tests are shown in Table 4.1q.

Table 4.1q Pulmonary function tests (1)

	Predicted	Actual	% Predicted
FEV₁ (L)	2.73	2.19	80
FVC (L)	3.98	2.58	65
FEV₁/FVC (%)		85	
TLC (L)	5.82	4.17	72
DLCO (mL/mmHg/minute)	25.3	7.2	28

a) Describe the preparation and conduct of basic spirometry *(6 marks)*
b) What is the meaning of the term 'FVC'? *(1 mark)*
c) What is the meaning of 'FEV₁/FVC ratio'? *(1 mark)*
d) What is the meaning and clinical relevance of DLCO? *(1 mark)*
e) What is the meaning of the term 'TLC'? *(1 mark)*
f) What do the pulmonary function test show? *(3 marks)*
g) Pathology within which part of the respiratory system would account for these results? *(1 mark)*

You are asked to assess another patient who has presented with breathlessness. Their pulmonary function tests are shown in Table 4.2q.

Table 4.2q Pulmonary function tests (2)

	Predicted	Actual	% Predicted
FEV₁ (L)	2.62	1.01	39
FVC (L)	3.19	2.33	73
FEV₁/FVC (%)		44	
TLC (L)	4.99	5.99	122
DLCO (mL/mmHg/minute)	22.3	20.4	91

h) What do these pulmonary function tests show? *(2 marks)*
i) What differential diagnoses would account for these results? *(2 marks)*
j) How is spirometry used to grade the severity of chronic obstructive pulmonary disease (COPD)? *(1 mark)*
k) What threshold value of FEV₁ defines COPD as 'very severe'? *(1 mark)*

Answers

a) Describe the preparation and conduct of basic spirometry *(6 marks)*
- Preparation:
  - Advise the patient to not smoke for 24 hours prior to testing, and avoid exercise or a large meal immediately prior to the test
  - Record the patient's age, ethnicity, height, and weight for calculation of predicted values
- Equipment:
  - Disposable one-way mouthpiece, nose clip, and bacterial and viral filters
  - Spirometer
- Patient instructions:
  - In a sitting position, ask the patient to breathe in to maximal inspiration, create a tight seal around the mouthpiece, and blow into the device as forcibly and for as long as possible
  - A minimum of three technically acceptable recordings are taken out of a maximum of eight permitted attempts. The 'best result' for each parameter is recorded

b) What is the meaning of the term 'FVC'? *(1 mark)*
- Forced vital capacity is the total volume exhaled during a forced expiration from maximal inspiration to maximal expiration

c) What is the meaning of 'FEV_1/FVC ratio'? *(1 mark)*
- The proportion of the forced vital capacity expelled during the first second

d) What is the meaning and clinical relevance of DLCO? *(1 mark)*
- Lung diffusion capacity for carbon monoxide is a surrogate estimate of the ability for oxygen to pass from the alveolar to the red blood cell

e) What is the meaning of the term 'TLC'? *(1 mark)*
- Total lung capacity is the total volume of gas within the lung at maximal inspiration

f) What do the pulmonary function tests show? *(3 marks)*
- Reduced FEV_1 and FVC
- Normal to increased FEV_1/FVC ratio
- Reduced DLCO

g) Pathology within which part of the respiratory system would account for these results? *(1 mark)*
- The restrictive defect and severely reduced DLCO suggests pulmonary parenchymal disease e.g. pulmonary fibrosis or connective tissue diseases with pulmonary involvement

h) What do the pulmonary function tests show? *(2 marks)*
- Reduced FEV_1 with preserved FVC
- Reduced FEV_1/FVC ratio (<0.7)

i) What differential diagnoses would account for the results? *(2 marks)*

(1 mark per diagnosis to a maximum of 2)
- Asthma
- Chronic obstructive pulmonary disease
- Bronchiectasis

j) How is spirometry used to grade the severity of chronic obstructive pulmonary disease (COPD)? *(1 mark)*
- The severity of COPD is graded by the percentage predicted FEV_1

k) What threshold value of FEV_1 defines COPD as 'very severe'? (1 mark)
- <30% predicted

Further reading

British Thoracic Society (UK). A guide to performing quality assured diagnostic spirometry. 2013. Available at: https://www.brit-thoracic.org.uk/media/70454/spirometry_e-guide_2013.pdf [accessed 5 March 2017].

Liang B-M, Lam DCL, Feng Y-L. Clinical applications of lung function tests: a revisit. *Respirology* 2012;17:611–619.

National Institute for Health and Care Excellence (NICE). Chronic obstructive airways disease in over 16s: diagnosis and management. NICE Clinical Guideline [101]. 2010. Available at: https://www.nice.org.uk/guidance/cg101 [accessed 5 March 2017].

Pellegrino R, Viegi G, Brusasco V, Crapo R O, Burgos F, Casaburi R, et al. Interpretive strategies for lung function tests. *European Respiratory Journal* 2005;26:948–968.

UK syllabus references 2.2, 2.7, 3.2.
CoBaTrICE domains 2, 5.

OSCE 4 station 6—data

Questions

A 54-year-old man with a background history of alcohol abuse has been admitted to the critical care unit with severe hypokalaemia (serum potassium 1.7 mmol/L (normal range: 3.5–5.3 mmol/L)).

The patient complains of rapid weight loss, chronic upper abdominal pain, and vomiting. He has moderate epigastric tenderness and appears dehydrated.

Blood analysis shows (normal ranges in brackets):

- Sodium 130 mmol/L (135–145 mmol/L)
- Chloride 82 mmol/L (95–105 mmol/L)
- Urea 12.3 mmol/L (2.5–6.7 mmol/L)
- Creatinine 118 µmol/L (70–100 µmol/L)
- Serum bicarbonate 37 mmol/L (24–30 mmol/L)

a) What is the most likely diagnosis? *(1 mark)*
b) What is the cause of the hypochloraemic alkalosis seen in gastric outlet obstruction? *(1 mark)*
c) What is the cause of hypokalaemia in gastric outlet obstruction? *(1 mark)*
d) Why might gastric outlet obstruction cause acute kidney injury? *(1 mark)*
e) What are the two most common causes of gastric outlet obstruction in adults? *(2 marks)*
f) What urinary acid–base changes are classically seen in gastric outlet obstruction? *(2 marks)*
g) What electrocardiogram changes are seen in severe hypokalaemia? *(6 marks)*

An upper gastrointestinal endoscopy shows the cause of the obstruction to be a localized gastric tumour. A non-emergency gastrectomy is planned.

h) Aside from correction of the electrolyte abnormalities, what two key areas of this patient's medical management should be addressed prior to surgery? *(2 marks)*
i) How might the risk of refeeding syndrome be reduced? *(4 marks)*

Answers

a) What is the most likely diagnosis? *(1 mark)*
   - Gastric outlet obstruction
b) What is the cause of the hypochloraemic alkalosis seen in gastric outlet obstruction? *(1 mark)*
   - Vomiting resulting in the loss of hydrogen and chloride ions
c) What is the cause of hypokalaemia in gastric outlet obstruction? *(1 mark)*
   - Dehydration results in activation of the renin–angiotensin system, resulting in renal loss of potassium
d) Why might gastric outlet obstruction cause acute kidney injury? *(1 mark)*
   - Hypovolaemia resulting in prerenal acute tubular necrosis
e) What are the two most common causes of gastric outlet obstruction in adults? *(2 marks)*
   - Gastric carcinoma
   - Peptic ulcer disease
f) What urinary acid–base changes are classically seen in gastric outlet obstruction? *(2 marks)*
   - Urine pH is initially high due to renal bicarbonate loss
   - Later, a 'paradoxical aciduria' develops as hydrogen ions are exchanged for sodium ions to maintain the circulating volume
g) What electrocardiogram changes are seen in severe hypokalaemia? *(6 marks)*
   - U waves
   - T-wave flattening and inversion
   - ST depression
   - Prolongation of the PR interval
   - Increased amplitude and width of the P wave
   - Arrhythmias
h) Aside from correction of the electrolyte abnormalities, what two key areas of this patient's medical management should be addressed prior to surgery? *(2 marks)*
   - Nutritional support
   - Management of alcohol withdrawal
i) How might the risk of refeeding syndrome be reduced? *(4 marks)*
   - Intravenous thiamine
   - Correcting potassium, phosphate, and magnesium prior to commencing feed
   - Starting feed at no more than 50% of calculated requirements
   - Frequent monitoring and correction of electrolyte abnormalities

Further reading

Koop AH, Palmer WC, Stancampiano FF. Gastric outlet obstruction: a red flag, potentially manageable. *Cleveland Clinic Journal of Medicine* 2019;86:345–353.

FFICM syllabus references 1.1, 2.3, 2.5, 2.8, 3.1, 3.2, 3.4, 3.7, 4.4, 4.8, 6.1.
CoBaTrICE domains 2, 3, 6.

OSCE 4 station 7—data

Questions

A 52-year-old man is failing to wean after a long period of invasive ventilation. He has generalized limb weakness, decreased muscular tone, and areflexia.

a) What pathologies cause intensive care unit-associated weakness (ICUAW)? *(3 marks)*
b) Which groups of medications are commonly associated with ICUAW? *(4 marks)*
c) What features of weakness are used to diagnose ICUAW? *(5 marks)*

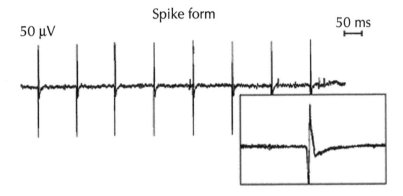

Spike form

50 µV

50 ms

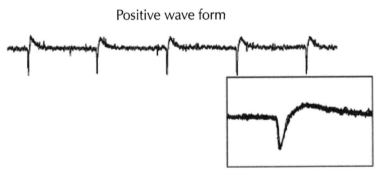

Positive wave form

Figure 4.5 Investigation

Reproduced from *Clinical Neurophysiology, Fourth Edition*, Rubin DI and Daube JR, Figure 24.18, Oxford University Press. © 2016 Mayo Foundation for Medical Education and Research. Reproduced with permission of the Licensor through PLSclear

Look at Figure 4.5.

d) What investigation has been performed? *(1 mark)*

e) Complete Table 4.3q to describe the results of investigations seen in critical illness polyneuropathy (CIP) and critical illness myopathy (CIM) *(6 marks)*

Table 4.3q Results of investigations in critical illness polyneuropathy and critical illness myopathy

Investigation	CIP	CIM
Nerve conduction studies	Reduced motor and _____ sensory action potential amplitudes, normal conduction velocity	Reduced motor and _____ sensory action potential amplitudes, normal conduction velocity
Electromyography	Spontaneous fibrillation potentials with _____ duration, _____ amplitude motor unit potentials	Spontaneous fibrillation potentials with _ _____ duration, _____ amplitude motor unit potentials

f) Which drug should be avoided in patients with ICUAW? *(1 mark)*

Answers

a) What pathologies cause intensive care unit-associated weakness (ICUAW)? *(3 marks)*
   - Critical illness polyneuropathy
   - Critical illness myopathy
   - Critical illness neuromyopathy

b) Which groups of medications are commonly associated with ICUAW? *(4 marks)*
   - Corticosteroids
   - Neuromuscular blocking agents
   - High-dose vasopressors
   - Aminoglycosides

c) What features of weakness are used to diagnose ICUAW? *(5 marks)*
   - Onset—weakness developing after the onset of critical illness
   - Distribution—generalized, symmetrical, flaccid weakness, generally sparing the cranial nerves
   - Duration—noted on more than two occasions separated by >24 hours
   - Effects—dependence on mechanical ventilation or failure to mobilize
   - Aetiology—causes of weakness not related to the underlying critical illness have been excluded

d) What investigation has been performed? *(1 mark)*
   - Electromyography

e) Complete Table 4.3a to describe the results of investigations seen in critical illness polyneuropathy (CIP) and critical illness myopathy (CIM) *(6 marks)*

Table 4.3a Results of investigations in critical illness polyneuropathy and critical illness myopathy

Investigation	CIP	CIM
Nerve conduction studies	Reduced motor and *reduced* sensory action potential amplitudes, normal conduction velocity	Reduced motor and *normal* sensory action potential amplitudes, normal conduction velocity
Electromyography	Spontaneous fibrillation potentials with *long* duration, *high* amplitude motor unit potentials	Spontaneous fibrillation potentials with *short* duration, *low* amplitude motor unit potentials

f) Which drug should be avoided in patients with ICUAW? *(1 mark)*
   - Suxamethonium

Further reading

Appleton R, Kinsella J. Intensive care unit-acquired weakness. *Continuing Education in Anaesthesia Critical Care & Pain* 2012:12:62–66.

FFICM syllabus references 2.2, 3.6.
CoBaTrICE domains 2.

OSCE 4 station 8—data

Questions

Look at Figure 4.6.

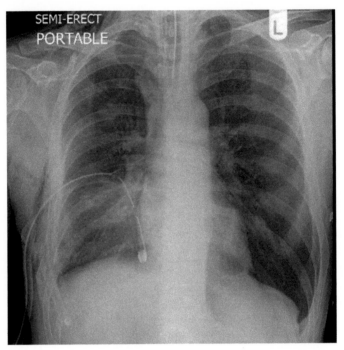

Figure 4.6 Chest X-ray

a) What findings can be seen on this chest X-ray? *(7 marks)*
b) Describe the anatomical borders of the 'triangle of safety', used to identify a safe site for intercostal drain insertion *(4 marks)*
c) What anatomical landmark describes the insertion point of an anterior apical chest drain? *(1 mark)*
d) What is a flail chest? *(3 marks)*
e) What are the proposed benefits of surgical rib fixation for flail chest? *(4 marks)*
f) What long-term complication is associated with successful surgical rib fixation? *(1 mark)*

Answers

a) What findings can be seen on this chest X-ray? *(7 marks)*
- Endotracheal tube
- Intercostal drain
- Nasogastric tube present in the left lung
- Surgical emphysema
- Multiple rib fractures of the right hemithorax
- Right lower zone opacification
- Healed rib fractures left hemithorax

b) Describe the anatomical borders of the 'triangle of safety', used to identify a safe site for intercostal drain insertion *(4 marks)*
- Anterior—lateral border of pectoralis major
- Posterior—lateral border of latissimus dorsi
- Inferior—horizontal line from the nipple (or fifth intercostal space)
- Superior—base of axilla

c) What anatomical landmark describes the insertion point of an anterior apical chest drain? *(1 mark)*
- Second intercostal space, mid-clavicular line

d) What is a flail chest? *(3 marks)*
- Fractures of two or more adjacent ribs ...
- ... in two or more places
- ... resulting in paradoxical chest movement

e) What are the proposed benefits of surgical rib fixation for flail chest? *(4 marks)*

(1 mark per benefit to a maximum of 4)
- Improved analgesia
- Reduced risk of pneumonia
- Reduced duration of mechanical ventilation
- Reduced critical care and hospital stay
- Decreased chest wall deformity
- Faster medium- to long-term recovery of respiratory function

f) What long-term complication is associated with successful surgical rib fixation? *(1 mark)*
- Chronic pain

Further reading

Havelock T, Teoh R, Laws D, Gleeson F. Pleural procedures and thoracic ultrasound: British Thoracic Society pleural disease guideline 2010. *Thorax* 2010;65(Suppl 2):ii61–ii76.

National Institute for Health and Care Excellence. Insertion of metal rib reinforcements to stabilise a flail chest wall. Interventional procedures guidance [IPG361]. 2010. Available at: https://www.nice.org.uk/guidance/ipg361 [accessed 26 February 2018].

FFICM syllabus references 1.5, 2.2, 2.6, 3.8, 7.2.
CoBaTrICE domains 2, 5.

OSCE 4 station 9—data

Questions

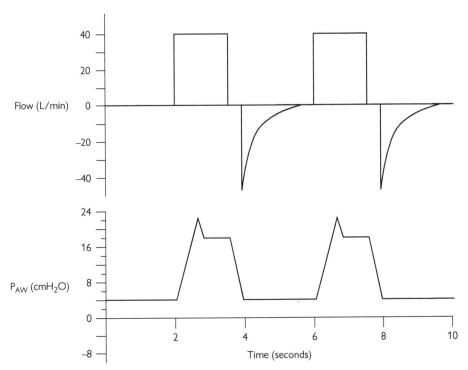

Figure 4.7 Ventilator waveforms

Look at Figure 4.7.

a) What do these ventilator waveforms show? *(4 marks)*
b) What is the …? *(5 marks)*
   • Positive end expiratory pressure (PEEP)
   • Peak airway pressure
   • Plateau airway pressure
   • Inspiratory:expiratory ratio
   • Respiratory rate
c) What mechanism would cause an increase in the plateau pressure? *(1 mark)*
d) What mechanism would cause an increase in the peak airway pressure but not of the plateau pressure? *(1 mark)*
e) What are the key features of assist control ventilation? *(3 marks)*

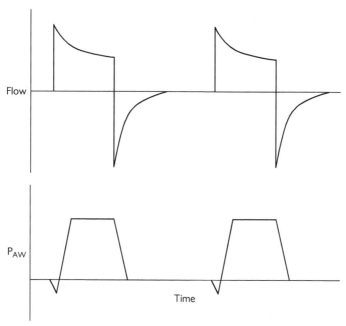

Figure 4.8 Ventilator waveforms

Look at Figure 4.8.

f) What do these waveforms show? *(2 marks)*

g) What determines the end of inspiration with supported ventilation breaths? *(1 mark)*

h) What triggers are used for ventilators to support a patient-initiated breath? *(2 marks)*

i) A patient who is receiving pressure support has a trigger setting of 0.2 L per minute. The ventilator is attempting to support a respiratory frequency of 90 breaths per minute despite the patient having a respiratory rate of 22 breaths per minute. What is the most likely cause? *(1 mark)*

Answers

a) What do these ventilator waveforms show? *(4 marks)*
   - A constant flow ...
   - ... time cycled ...
   - ... mandatory ...
   - ... volume-controlled breath

b) What is the ...? *(5 marks)*
   - Positive end-expiratory pressure (PEEP): 4 cmH$_2$O
   - Peak airway pressure: 22 cmH$_2$O
   - Plateau airway pressure: 18 cmH$_2$O
   - Inspiratory:expiratory ratio: 1:1
   - Respiratory rate: 15 breaths per minute

c) What mechanism would cause an increase in the plateau pressure? *(1 mark)*
   - A reduction in compliance

d) What mechanism would cause an increase in the peak airway pressure but not of the plateau pressure? *(1 mark)*
   - An increase in airway resistance

e) What are the key features of assist control ventilation? *(3 marks)*
   - Ventilation occurs at or above a set minimum rate
   - Ventilation can be initiated by the patient or the ventilator
   - Patient- and machine-triggered breaths are identical

f) What do these waveforms show? *(2 marks)*
   - Spontaneous respiration, with pressure support

g) What determines the end of inspiration with supported ventilation breaths? *(1 mark)*
   - A reduction in inspiratory flow by a preset proportion

h) What triggers are used for ventilators to support a patient-initiated breath? *(2 marks)*
   - A flow rate of a preset value generated by the patient
   - A reduction in pressure below a preset value in the ventilator circuit

i) A patient who is receiving pressure support has a trigger setting of 0.2 L per minute. The ventilator is attempting to support a respiratory frequency of 90 breaths per minute despite the patient having a respiratory rate of 22 breaths per minute. What is the most likely cause? *(1 mark)*
   - The ventilator is sensing the patient's heart beat as the start of a spontaneous breath. Increasing the trigger would resolve the issue

Notes

Ventilator terminology can be a source of great confusion because of the number of 'modes' available, and the nomenclature used by different ventilator manufacturers. In essence, however, there are only so many variables that make up a ventilator mode (cycling, pressure vs volume controlled, how flow is delivered, how and when the patient can breathe, etc.), so by looking at them in terms of these features you will gain the understanding that will allow you to answer questions such as this from 'first principles'.

Further reading

Kreit JW. *Mechanical Ventilation*. Oxford: Oxford University Press; 2013.

FFICM syllabus references 2.7, 3.8, 4.6.
CoBaTrICE domains 2, 4.

OSCE 4 station 10—data

Questions

a) What is the purpose of a ventricular assist device (VAD)? *(1 mark)*

b) How can VADs be classified? *(4 marks)*

c) Where do left ventricular assist devices (LVADs) and right ventricular assist devices (RVADs) take blood from and eject blood into? *(4 marks)*

d) What are the indications for use of a VAD? *(3 marks)*

e) Is there an evidence base for the insertion of LVADs in patients with end-stage heart failure? *(2 marks)*

f) What problem does a LVAD pose when inserting a peripheral arterial cannula? *(1 mark)*

g) What are the potential complications of VAD insertion? *(5 marks)*

Answers

a) What is the purpose of a ventricular assist device (VAD)? *(1 mark)*
  - To partially support or entirely replace the function of the left or right ventricle
b) How can VADs be classified? *(4 marks)*
  - Ventricle(s) being supported—left, right, biventricular
  - Mechanism—pusher plate (pulsatile), axial rotary (non-pulsatile)
  - Location—extracorporeal, paracorporeal, intracorporeal
  - Drive train—pneumatic, electrical, magnetic
c) Where do left ventricular assist devices (LVADs) and right ventricular assist devices (RVADs) take blood from and eject blood into? *(4 marks)*
  - A LVAD takes blood from the left ventricle and ...
  - ... usually ejects into the ascending or descending aorta
  - A RVAD takes blood from the right ventricle and ...
  - ... ejects into the pulmonary artery
d) What are the indications for use of a VAD? *(3 marks)*
  - Bridge to recovery, e.g. myocarditis, post-transplant reperfusion or rejection syndromes, post-cardiotomy low cardiac output
  - Bridge to transplant, i.e. progressive heart failure despite maximal medical management
  - Destination (permanent) therapy, i.e. patients in whom transplantation is required but contraindicated
e) Is there an evidence base for the insertion of LVADs in patients with end-stage heart failure? *(2 marks)*
  - Yes
  - The REMATCH trial compared permanent LVAD treatment with best medical management in patients with end-stage heart failure who were ineligible for transplant. It demonstrated a reduction in 1-year mortality with permanent LVAD treatment
f) What problem does an LVAD pose when inserting a peripheral arterial cannula? *(1 mark)*
  - Many of the devices are continuous flow devices. These patients will not have normal pulsatile flow so arterial line insertion is more difficult
g) What are the potential complications of VAD insertion? *(5 marks)*

  (1 mark per complication to a maximum of 5)
  - Acute:
    * Haemorrhage (VADs require systemic anticoagulation)
    * Air embolus
    * Right ventricular failure (common after LVAD insertion; up to 30% will subsequently need RVAD support)
    * Cannula obstruction
    * Haemolysis
    * Arrhythmias
    * Right-to-left shunting through a patent foramen ovale (LVAD)
    * Multiple organ failure
  - Chronic:
    * Thrombus formation/haemorrhage
    * Stroke
    * Infection
    * Valve failure
    * Device failure

Further reading

Tubaro M, Vranckx P, Price S, Vrints C. *The ESC Textbook of Intensive and Acute Cardiovascular Care*, 2nd Edition. Oxford: Oxford University Press; 2015.

Webb A, Angus D, Finfer S, Gattinoni L, Singer M. *Oxford Textbook of Critical Care*, 2nd Edition. Oxford: Oxford University Press; 2016.

FFICM syllabus references 3.1, 3.2, 3.3, 4.5, 5.8, 6.2.
CoBaTrICE domains 3, 4, 5, 6.

OSCE 4 station 11—data

Questions

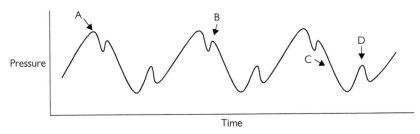

Figure 4.9 CVP waveform

Look at the central venous pressure (CVP) waveform shown in Figure 4.9.

a) What do the labels A, B, C, and D on the waveform represent? *(4 marks)*
b) What changes in the CVP waveform would be seen in a patient with significant tricuspid regurgitation? *(1 mark)*
c) Which arrhythmias can cause cannon A waves in the CVP waveform? *(4 marks)*

A patient presents to the critical care unit with hypoxaemia related to pulmonary arterial hypertension (PAH).

d) How is pulmonary hypertension defined? *(2 marks)*
e) How can echocardiography help in the diagnostic workup of a patient with suspected PAH? *(4 marks)*
f) What pulmonary vasodilators are available to treat PAH in the intensive care unit? *(5 marks)*

Answers

a) What do the labels A, B, C, and D on the waveform represent? *(4 marks)*
   - A—atrial contraction (A wave)
   - B—doming of tricuspid valve into right atrium (C wave)
   - C—atrial relaxation (X decent)
   - D—atrial filling before tricuspid valve opening (V wave)
b) What changes in the CVP waveform would be seen in a patient with significant tricuspid regurgitation? *(1 mark)*
   - An enlarged V wave that obliterates the X decent, creating a 'CV wave'
c) Which arrhythmias can cause cannon A waves in the CVP waveform? *(4 marks)*
   - Complete heart block
   - Ventricular tachycardia
   - Junctional rhythm
   - Atrioventricular nodal re-entry tachycardia
d) How is pulmonary hypertension defined? *(2 marks)*
   - Mean pulmonary artery pressure of >25 mmHg ...
   - ... at rest as assessed by right heart catheterization
e) How can echocardiography help in the diagnostic workup of a patient with suspected PAH? *(4 marks)*
   - Assessment of ventricular function
   - Exclusion of significant left-to-right shunts
   - Estimation of pulmonary artery pressure
   - Assessment of valve function
f) What pulmonary vasodilators are available to treat PAH in the intensive care unit? *(5 marks)*

   (1 mark per answer to a maximum of 5)
   - Phosphodiesterase-5 inhibitors
   - Endothelin receptor antagonists
   - Prostaglandins
   - Inhaled nitric oxide
   - Soluble guanylate cyclase stimulators
   - Calcium channel blockers

Notes

The CVP waveform and its pathological variations are exam favourites.

FFICM syllabus references 2.7, 3.1, 4.4.
CoBaTrICE domains 2, 3.

OSCE 4 station 12—equipment

Questions

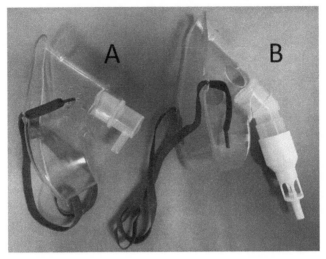

Figure 4.10 Oxygen masks

Look at Figure 4.10.

a) Regarding mask A, what factors affect the fraction of inspired oxygen? *(4 marks)*

b) Why does mask A have side holes? *(2 marks)*

c) What is mask B called? *(1 mark)*

d) How does mask B provide a fixed fraction of inspired oxygen? *(3 marks)*

e) The outcomes of which adult diseases might be worsened by hyperoxic therapy? *(4 marks)*

f) By what mechanisms might hyperoxia cause harm in acute myocardial infarction? *(2 marks)*

g) What are the symptoms of oxygen toxicity? *(4 marks)*

Answers

a) Regarding mask A, what factors affect the fraction of inspired oxygen? *(4 marks)*
  - Peak inspiratory flow rate
  - Respiratory rate
  - Oxygen flow rate
  - Mask fit

b) Why does mask A have side holes? *(2 marks)*
  - To entrain ambient air when the inspiratory flow exceeds oxygen flow
  - To allow expired gases to be flushed out by the fresh gas flow

c) What is mask B called? *(1 mark)*
  - High air flow oxygen enrichment (HAFOE) or venturi mask

d) How does mask B provide a fixed fraction of inspired oxygen? *(3 marks)*
  - As oxygen flows through a constriction in the nozzle, the resultant negative entrains ambient air (Bernoulli effect)
  - The combined gas flow exceeds the peak inspiratory flow rate, ensuring ambient air is not entrained into the mixture
  - The size of the nozzle aperture determines the quantity of entrained ambient air for a given oxygen flow rate, ensuring a fixed fraction of inspired oxygen

e) The outcomes of which adult diseases in might be worsened by hyperoxic therapy? *(4 marks)*

  (1 mark per answer to a maximum of 4)
  - Lung diseases featuring a hypoxic respiratory drive
  - Acute stroke
  - Acute myocardial infarction
  - Acute lung injury
  - Severe head injury
  - Post-cardiac arrest syndrome

f) By what mechanisms might hyperoxia cause harm in acute myocardial infarction? *(2 marks)*
  - Free radical production
  - Coronary vasoconstriction

g) What are the symptoms of oxygen toxicity? *(4 marks)*

  (1 mark per answer to a maximum of 4)
  - Tunnel vision
  - Tinnitus
  - Nausea
  - Vertigo
  - Behavioural changes (anxiety, irritability, confusion)
  - Facial numbness
  - Twitching of the face or small muscles of the hands
  - Seizures
  - Retrosternal chest pain
  - Dyspnoea
  - Coughing

FFICM syllabus references 1.1, 2.7, 3.1, 3.2, 3.8, 4.1, 5.1.
CoBaTrICE domains 1, 3, 4.

OSCE 4 station 13—equipment

Questions

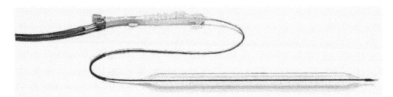

Figure 4.11 Medical device
Reproduced from *Cardiac Catheterization and Coronary Intervention*, Mitchell ARJ et al., Figure 8.2. © 2008 Oxford University Press. Reproduced with permission of the Licensor through PLSclear

Look at Figure 4.11.

a) What is this piece of equipment? *(1 mark)*
b) What are the primary functions of an intra-aortic balloon pump (IABP)? *(1 mark)*
c) What is the balloon inflated with and why? *(2 marks)*
d) In an adult, where should the tip of the balloon lie when correctly positioned? *(1 mark)*
e) What are potential clinical indications for the use of an IABP? *(3 marks)*
f) What conditions would be contraindications for IABP use? *(4 marks)*
g) What are the effects of a correctly working IABP on left ventricular afterload, preload, ejection fraction, and wall stress *(4 marks)*
h) What are the potential complications of IABP use? *(4 marks)*

Answers

a) What is this piece of equipment? *(1 mark)*
   - Intra-aortic balloon catheter
b) What are the primary functions of an intra-aortic balloon pump (IABP)? *(1 mark)*
   - To increase myocardial oxygen supply and decrease myocardial oxygen demand
c) What is the balloon inflated with and why? *(2 marks)*
   - Helium gas
   - Helium has a low viscosity, allowing it to travel quickly through the long connecting tubes. Also, the risk of causing an embolism if the balloon ruptures is lower than with air
d) In an adult, where should the tip of the balloon lie when correctly positioned? *(1 mark)*
   - In the descending thoracic aorta approximately 2 cm distal to the origin of the left subclavian artery
e) What are potential clinical indications for the use of an IABP? *(3 marks)*

   (1 mark per answer to a maximum of 3)
   - Refractory left ventricular failure
   - Cardiogenic shock
   - Refractory unstable angina
   - Acute myocardial infarction
   - Acute mitral regurgitation and ventricular septal defect post myocardial infarction
   - Weaning from cardiopulmonary bypass
   - Cardiac surgery
   - Cardiac support for high-risk general surgery and angioplasty
   - Sepsis
   - Infants and children with complex cardiac anomalies
f) What conditions would be contraindications for IABP use? *(4 marks)*

   (1 mark per answer to a maximum of 4)
   - Absolute:
     - Severe aortic regurgitation
     - Aortic dissection
     - Aortic stents
     - End-stage heart disease with no prospect of recovery
   - Relative:
     - Severe peripheral vascular disease
     - Aortic aneurysm
     - Major arterial reconstructive surgery
     - Sepsis
     - Tachyarrhythmias
g) What are the effects of a correctly working IABP on left ventricular afterload, preload, ejection fraction, and wall stress *(4 marks)*
   - Reduced afterload
   - Reduced preload
   - Increased ejection fraction
   - Reduced wall stress
h) What are the potential complications of IABP use? *(4 marks)*

   (1 mark per answer to a maximum of 4)
   - Vascular:
     - Limb ischaemia
     - Femoral artery thrombosis

- ◆ Peripheral embolization
- ◆ Femoral vein cannulation
- ◆ Arterial injury
- ◆ Arteriovenous fistula formation
- ◆ False aneurysm
- ● Balloon related:
  - ◆ Perforation
  - ◆ Rupture
  - ◆ Incorrect positioning
  - ◆ Gas embolization
  - ◆ Entrapment
- ● Other:
  - ◆ Haemorrhage
  - ◆ Visceral ischaemia
  - ◆ Infection
  - ◆ Compartment syndrome
  - ◆ Thrombocytopenia

Notes

The examiner doesn't need all contradictions, complications, etc. for you to achieve full marks, so if they move you along mid answer that might not always be such a bad thing!

Further reading

Krishna M, Zacharowski K. Principles of intra-aortic balloon pump counterpulsation. *Continuing Education in Anaesthesia Critical Care & Pain* 2009;9:24–28.

FFICM syllabus references 1.1, 2.7, 3.1, 3.3, 4.5, 6.1, 6.2.
CoBaTrICE domains 1, 4, 5, 6.

OSCE 5

OSCE 5 station 1—professionalism

Questions

Eric has been a patient on the intensive care unit for 7 days and the team have decided that insertion of a percutaneous tracheostomy would be in his best medical interests. Eric does not have capacity to consent for the procedure. You are about to discuss the procedure with Eric's wife. She asks:

a) 'What is a tracheostomy?' *(3 marks)*
b) 'Why do you think it would be helpful?' *(3 marks)*
c) 'Are there any risks?' *(6 marks)*
d) 'What about the consent form? Surely Eric isn't well enough to sign it?' *(4 marks)*

Answers

a) 'What is a tracheostomy?' *(3 marks)*
- A tracheostomy is a breathing tube inserted into the front of Eric's neck allowing the removal of the breathing tube in his mouth
- The tracheostomy should be temporary
- Insertion of the tracheostomy is a surgical procedure performed on the intensive care unit

b) 'Why do you think it would be helpful?' *(3 marks)*
- To increase comfort (removal of sedation, aiding communication, and allowing earlier resumption of oral diet)
- To aid gradual removal of the ventilator (weaning)
- To help with secretion clearance

c) 'Are there any risks?' *(6 marks)*

(1 mark per potential complication to a maximum of 6)
- Bleeding
- Collapsed lung
- Problems with oxygen levels or blood pressure or the heart during the procedure
- Accidental damage to other structures in the neck such as the food pipe
- Wound infection or problems with healing
- Scarring, narrowing of the windpipe
- Changes in the strength or pitch of the voice
- Possibility of blood transfusion or emergency surgery
- Risk of death (<0.2%)

d) 'What about the consent form? Surely Eric isn't well enough to sign it?' *(4 marks)*

- Ensure that Eric does not have a lasting power of attorney for healthcare
- Explain the concepts of capacity and best interests
- State that consent is provided by a health professional
- Explain that the consent process includes consideration of the views of family members/significant others and of any previously expressed wishes

General communication *(4 marks)*
Marks awarded for behaviours such as the following:

- Eye contact, introduces self, and body language
- Pace and volume of speech
- Demonstrates empathy and addresses questions, concerns, and anxieties
- Offers clear explanations
- Avoids medical jargon

Notes

This question relates to capacity as applied in England and Wales. For the purposes of the UK FFICM examination, you would not be penalized for applying the law as it applies in Scotland or Northern Ireland.

FFICM syllabus references 4.6, 7.1, 7.4, 11.8, 12.1, 12.4, 12.12.
CoBaTrICE domains 5, 12.

OSCE 5 station 2—resuscitation

Questions

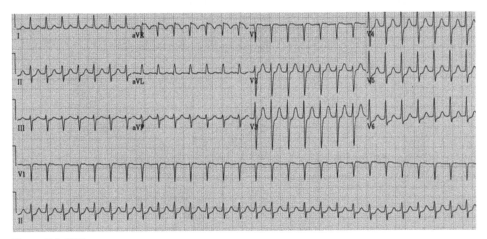

Figure 5.1 ECG

Reproduced from *Essential Revision Notes for the Cardiology KBA*, Khavandi A, Figure 7.5. © 2014 Oxford University Press. Reproduced with permission of the Licensor through PLSclear

You are called to the coronary care unit to review a patient with tachycardia. The patient is 45 years old and was admitted 12 hours previously, following an episode of tachycardia and dizziness.

Your examination findings are as follows:

- Respiratory rate 18 breaths per minute, chest auscultation is normal, saturations 98% on room air
- Pulse 200 beats per minute (bpm), blood pressure (BP) 110/70 mmHg
- Glasgow Coma Scale score 15/15

Biochemistry results from 2 hours ago are within normal limits.

Look at Figure 5.1.

a) How can this clinical picture be described? *(1 mark)*
b) What adverse features of tachycardia would you specifically look for? *(4 marks)*
c) How do the Resuscitation Council (UK) define 'shock' in their guidelines? *(3 marks)*
d) How would you treat this patient's tachycardia? *(2 marks)*
e) What are the contraindications to treatment with adenosine? *(3 marks)*

The nurse alerts you to a change in the patient's observations.

- Respiratory rate 20 breaths minute, saturations 95% on room air
- Heart rate 280 bpm, BP 70/40 mmHg
- Glasgow Coma Scale score E1, V1, M2

f) What treatment is now required? *(2 marks)*
g) How much energy should be delivered with the first shock when performing synchronized direct current (DC) cardioversion for a regular narrow complex tachycardia? *(1 mark)*
h) You deliver three shocks but there is no improvement in the patient's condition. What would you do next? *(4 marks)*

Answers

a) How can this clinical picture be described? *(1 mark)*
  - Haemodynamically stable narrow complex tachycardia

b) What adverse features of tachycardia would you specifically look for? *(4 marks)*
  - Shock
  - Syncope
  - Myocardial ischaemia
  - Heart failure

c) How do the Resuscitation Council (UK) define 'shock' in their guidelines? *(3 marks)*
  - Systolic blood pressure <90 mmHg
  - Poor peripheral perfusion
  - Altered cognition

d) How would you treat this patient's tachycardia? *(2 marks)*
  - Vagal manoeuvres
  - Adenosine 6 mg, increasing to 12 mg if required

e) What are the contraindications to treatment with adenosine? *(3 marks)*

  (1 mark per contraindication to a maximum of 3)
  - Asthma or chronic obstructive pulmonary disease
  - Decompensated heart failure
  - Long QT syndrome
  - Second- or third-degree heart block
  - Sick sinus syndrome
  - Severe hypotension

f) What treatment is now required? *(2 marks)*
  - Synchronized ...
  - ... DC shock

g) How much energy should be delivered with the first shock when performing synchronized direct current (DC) cardioversion for a regular narrow complex tachycardia? *(1 mark)*
  - 70–120 J

h) You deliver three shocks but there is no improvement in the patient's condition. What would you do next? *(4 marks)*
  - Seek expert help
  - Give a loading dose of amiodarone—300 mg IV over 10–20 minutes
  - Repeat the synchronized shock
  - Give a maintenance dose of amiodarone—900 mg IV over 24 hours

Further reading

Resuscitation Council (UK). Adult tachycardia (with pulse) algorithm. 2015. Available at: https://www.resus.org.uk/resuscitation-guidelines/peri-arrest-arrhythmias/#tachycardia [accessed 11 June 2018].

FFICM syllabus references 1.1, 2.1, 2.2, 2.3, 2.7, 3.1, 5.11, 11.3, 12.2.
CoBaTrICE domains 1, 2, 3, 4, 5.

OSCE 5 station 3—data

Questions

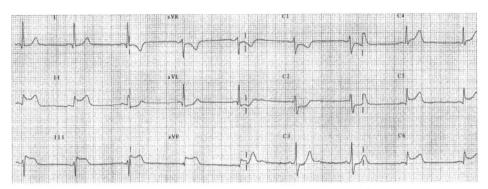

25mm/s   10mm/mV   F ∿ 0.05Hz–40Hz

Figure 5.2 Electrocardiogram (ECG)
Reproduced from *Oxford Handbook of Cardiac Nursing, Second Edition*, Olsen K, Figure 7.4. © 2014 Oxford University Press.
Reproduced with permission of the Licensor through PLSclear

A 59-year-old man is admitted to intensive care following an elective abdominal aortic aneurysm repair. He initially makes a good recovery but on day 3, while awaiting a ward bed, develops central crushing chest pain radiating to his left arm. He is clammy and breathless.

Look at Figure 5.2.

a) What abnormalities are shown on this electrocardiogram (ECG) and what is the diagnosis?
   (2 marks)
b) Name the coronary arteries most likely to cause the infarct territories shown in Table 5.1q
   (4 marks)

Table 5.1q Infarct territories

Infarct territory	Coronary artery
Anterior (V1–4)	
Inferior (II, II, aVF)	
Lateral (I, V5, V6)	
Posterior (V7–9)	

c) Under what circumstances should primary percutaneous intervention (PCI) be used as the preferred coronary reperfusion strategy for patients with acute ST elevation myocardial infarction (STEMI)? *(2 marks)*

d) State the mechanism of action for the antiplatelet agents listed in Table 5.2q *(3 marks)*

Table 5.2q Antiplatelet mechanisms of action

Drug(s)	Mechanism of action
Aspirin	
Clopidogrel, prasugrel, ticagrelor	
Tirofiban, abciximab	

The patient is reintubated and transferred to the angiography suite.

e) What are the challenges of providing critical care in an angiography suite? *(5 marks)*
f) What structural cardiac complications can occur acutely following a STEMI? *(4 marks)*

Answers

a) What abnormalities are shown on this electrocardiogram (ECG) and what is the diagnosis? *(2 marks)*
  - ST elevation in II, III, AVF, and V4–6
  - Inferolateral ST elevation myocardial infarction

b) Name the coronary arteries most likely to cause the infarct territories shown in Table 5.1a *(4 marks)*

Table 5.1a Infarct territories

Infarct territory	Coronary artery
Anterior (V1–4)	*Left anterior descending*
Inferior (II, II, aVF)	*Right coronary artery*
Lateral (I, V5, V6)	*Left circumflex*
Posterior (V7–9)	*Right coronary artery*

c) Under what circumstances should primary percutaneous intervention (PCI) be used as the preferred coronary reperfusion strategy for patients with acute ST elevation myocardial infarction (STEMI)? *(2 marks)*
  - Presentation within 12 hours of onset of symptoms and
  - Primary PCI can be delivered within 120 minutes of the time when fibrinolysis could have been administered

d) State the mechanism of action for the antiplatelet agents listed in Table 5.2a *(3 marks)*

Table 5.2a Antiplatelet mechanisms of action

Drug(s)	Mechanism of action
Aspirin	*Cyclooxygenase 1 (COX1) inhibitor*
Clopidogrel, prasugrel, ticagrelor	*ADP pathway or P2Y12 receptor inhibitors*
Tirofiban, abciximab	*Glycoprotein IIb/IIIa inhibitors*

e) What are the challenges of providing critical care in an angiography suite? *(5 marks)*
  - Equipment—availability, compatibility, familiarity, completion of safety checks
  - Staff—cardiology staff are not usually trained in critical care and may be unfamiliar with equipment
  - Procedure—darkened room, limited access and space, potential procedural unfamiliarity
  - Patient—positioning, potential instability
  - Anaesthetic technique—often limited by equipment available, different techniques may be required

f) What structural cardiac complications can occur following a STEMI? *(4 marks)*

(1 mark per complication to a maximum of 4)
- Ventricular free wall rupture
- Ventricular septal rupture
- Papillary muscle rupture
- Mitral valve regurgitation
- Left ventricular aneurysm

Further reading

Steg P, James S, Atar D, Badano L, Blomstrom-Lundqvist C, Crea F, et al. ESC Guidelines for the management of acute myocardial infarction in patients presenting with ST-segment elevation: The Task Force on the management of ST-segment elevation acute myocardial infarction of the European Society of Cardiology (ESC). *European Heart Journal* 2012;33:2569–2619.

FFICM syllabus references 1.1, 2.1, 2.2, 2.3, 2.7, 3.1, 3.3, 4.1, 6.1, 10.1, 12.2, 12.9, 12.11.
CoBaTrICE domains 1, 2, 3, 4, 6, 10.

OSCE 5 station 4—data

Questions

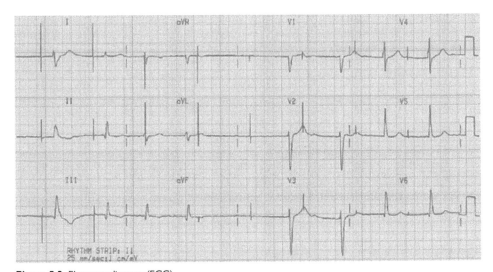

Figure 5.3 Electrocardiogram (ECG)

Reproduced from *Emergencies in Cardiology, Second Edition*, Myerson SG et al., Figure 21.44. © 2009 Oxford University Press. Reproduced with permission of the Licensor through PLSclear

You are asked to review a patient on the cardiac intensive care unit who has undergone an un-complicated elective aortic valve replacement. The patient's electrocardiogram (ECG) is shown in Figure 5.3.

a) What abnormalities are present on the ECG? *(3 marks)*

b) What is the difference between failure to pace and failure to capture? *(1 mark)*

c) What are the likely causes of failure to pace post cardiac surgery? *(2 marks)*

d) What are the potential causes of failure of capture following cardiac surgery? *(2 marks)*

e) What is the sensitivity (or pacing) threshold? *(1 mark)*

f) How would you determine the sensitivity threshold using a temporary pacing box? *(2 marks)*

g) What are the risks of incorrectly setting the sensitivity during temporary pacing? *(2 marks)*

h) What is the stimulation (or capture) threshold? *(1 mark)*

i) How would you determine the stimulation threshold using a temporary pacing box? *(2 marks)*

j) Having determined the sensitivity and stimulation thresholds, how would you set the sensitivity and output on the pacing box? *(2 marks)*

k) What are the benefits of having atrial as well as a ventricular epicardial pacing leads? *(2 marks)*

Answers

a) What abnormalities are present on the ECG? *(3 marks)*
   - Atrial fibrillation
   - Ventricular ectopic
   - Pacing spikes with failure to capture

b) What is the difference between failure to pace and failure to capture? *(1 mark for both points)*
   - Failure to pace is the absence of pacing when the native rate is slower than the set rate (there is no attempt to pace when there should be)
   - In failure to capture, pacing spikes are present but dissociated from ECG complexes (the attempt to pace is unsuccessful)

c) What are the likely causes of failure to pace post cardiac surgery? *(2 marks)*

   (1 mark per cause to a maximum of 2)
   - Lead disconnection or unstable connection at the pacing box
   - Lead malfunction
   - Battery depletion
   - Over sensing—electromagnetic or mechanical interference (e.g. shivering) interpreted as native electrical activity
   - Cross talk when dual chamber pacing—the atrial pacing spike is interpreted by the ventricular lead as native activity, inhibiting ventricular pacing
   - Inappropriate pacemaker settings

d) What are the potential causes of failure to capture following cardiac surgery? *(2 marks)*

   (1 mark per cause to a maximum of 2)
   - Pacing wire displacement
   - Inappropriate pacemaker settings
   - Change in resistance due to electrolyte derangement, medications, recent defibrillation, ischaemia, inflammation/fibrosis at the lead tip

e) What is the sensitivity (or pacing) threshold? *(1 mark)*
   - The voltage (mV) at which the pacemaker box senses native electrical activity

f) How would you determine the sensitivity threshold using a temporary pacing box? *(2 marks)*
   - Set the rate to 10 beats per minute below the native rate and reduce the output
   - Increase the sensitivity of the system by reducing the voltage to the minimum setting. Then slowly reduce the sensitivity by increasing the voltage until the sense indicator (e.g. sensing light) stops flashing. Finally, slowly increase the sensitivity again by reducing the voltage until the sense indicator flashes at the native rate. The value in mV at which this occurs is the sensitivity threshold

g) What are the risks of incorrectly setting the sensitivity during temporary pacing? *(2 marks)*
   - Insensitive pacing systems pose a risk of atrial or ventricular fibrillation if pacing is delivered late in the depolarization phase
   - Excessively sensitive systems may detect lower amplitude activity (i.e. T waves) causing inappropriate inhibition of pacing

h) What is the stimulation (or capture) threshold? *(1 mark)*
   - The minimum current required to trigger an action potential in the myocardium

i) How would you determine the stimulation threshold using a temporary pacing box? *(2 marks)*
   - Set the rate 10 beats per minute above the native rate
   - Set the output (mA) to minimum and slowly increase until sustained electrical capture is seen on the ECG

j) Having determined the sensitivity and stimulation thresholds, how would you set the sensitivity and output on the pacing box? *(2 marks)*

- Output—2–3 × the measured stimulation threshold
- Sensitivity—30–50% of the measured sensitivity threshold (or at 2 mV if there is no underlying native rhythm)

k) What are the benefits of having atrial as well as a ventricular epicardial pacing leads? *(2 marks)*

(1 mark per benefit to a maximum of 2)
- Prevention of atrial fibrillation
- Management of bradycardia
- Preservation of atrioventricular coordination

Notes

Your comfort with this question is likely to depend on your experience. The concepts are not inherently complicated but require a degree of understanding and thought.

Further reading

Reade MC. Review article: Temporary epicardial pacing after cardiac surgery: a practical review. Part 2: selection of epicardial pacing modes and troubleshooting. *Anaesthesia* 2007;62:364–373.

FFICM syllabus references 2.3, 3.1, 3.3, 4.5, 5.12, 6.2.
CoBaTrICE domains 2, 3, 4, 5.

OSCE 5 station 5—data

Questions

You are called to assist in the management of a 1-year-old child admitted with respiratory failure suspected to be caused by bronchiolitis. The child has had several brief apnoeic episodes requiring facemask ventilation by the paediatric team.

a) What is the principal causative pathogen in bronchiolitis? *(1 mark)*

b) What test is most commonly used to confirm respiratory syncytial virus (RSV) as the causative pathogen in bronchiolitis? *(1 mark)*

c) What groups of children are at a higher risk of severe disease? *(3 marks)*

d) What is the estimated the weight of a 1-year-old child? *(1 mark)*

e) What signs might be observed at the bedside suggesting the child has increased work of breathing? *(3 marks)*

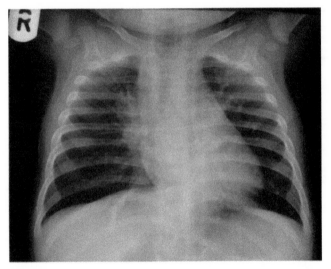

Figure 5.4 Chest X-ray
Reproduced from *Paediatric Radiology*, Johnson K et al., Figure 2.11. © 2009 Oxford University Press. Reproduced with permission of the Licensor through PLSclear

A chest X-ray is performed (Figure 5.4).

f) What abnormal features are shown on the X-ray? *(2 marks)*

A decision is made to intubate the child because of recurrent apnoea.

g) What are the anatomical differences between the infant and adult larynx? *(3 marks)*

Following intubation with a size 4 oral endotracheal tube, a significant leak is encountered.

h) What options are available to eliminate the leak? *(2 marks)*

A cuffed size 4.0 endotracheal tube is placed, eliminating the leak. Following this there is poor chest movement and high airway pressures.

i) What are the potential causes of this problem? *(4 marks)*

Answers

a) What is the principal causative pathogen in bronchiolitis? *(1 mark)*
  - Respiratory syncytial virus

b) What test is most commonly used to confirm respiratory syncytial virus (RSV) as the causative pathogen in bronchiolitis? *(1 mark)*
  - Immunofluorescence of nasopharyngeal aspirate

c) What groups of children are at a higher risk of severe disease? *(3 marks)*

  (1 mark per group to a maximum of 3)
  - Coexisting chronic lung disease
  - History of prematurity, especially <32 weeks
  - Immunodeficiency
  - Congenital heart disease
  - Age <3 months
  - Neuromuscular disorders
  - Passive smoke exposure

d) What is the estimated the weight of a 1-year-old child? *(1 mark)*
  - 10 kg

e) What signs might be observed at the bedside suggesting the child has increased work of breathing? *(3 marks)*

  (1 mark per sign to a maximum of 3)
  - Nasal flaring
  - Grunting
  - Intercostal and subcostal recession
  - Tachypnoea
  - Sweating

f) What abnormal features are shown on the X-ray? *(2 marks)*
  - Peribronchial thickening (cuffing)
  - Overinflated lung fields

g) What are the anatomical differences between the infant and adult larynx? *(3 marks)*
  - Infants have a high anterior larynx
  - Infants have a floppy, omega-shaped epiglottis
  - The subglottic area is the narrowest part in infants whereas in adults it is the glottic area

h) What options are available to eliminate the leak? *(2 marks)*
  - Reintubate with a larger uncuffed endotracheal tube
  - Reintubate with a same-sized cuffed endotracheal tube

i) What are the potential causes of this problem? *(4 marks)*

  (1 mark per cause to a maximum of 4)
  - Endobronchial tube placement
  - Kinked endotracheal tube
  - Airway obstruction from secretions
  - Pneumothorax
  - Dynamic hyperinflation from gas trapping
  - Gastric distension

Further reading

Meissner HC. Viral bronchiolitis in children. *New England Journal of Medicine* 2016;374:62–72.

FFICM syllabus reference 9.1.
CoBaTrICE domains 1, 2, 3, 4, 9.

OSCE 5 station 6—data

Questions

You are called to review a 17-year-old male in the emergency department who has been brought in by paramedics having been found unconscious in a park.

The findings of your initial assessment are:

A—patent with an oropharyngeal airway

B—SpO$_2$ 100% (15 L oxygen via a non-rebreathe mask). Respiratory rate 24 breaths per minute. Chest clear on auscultation

C—heart rate 115 beats per minute, blood pressure 100/50 mmHg, capillary refill time 4 seconds centrally

D—Glasgow Coma Scale score 9/15 (E2, V2, M5)

E—temperature 35.0°C. Clothes stained with vomit but no signs of external injury

An arterial blood gas (ABG) analysis shows (normal ranges in brackets):

- pH 7.23 (7.35–7.45)
- PCO$_2$ 3.8 kPa (4.7–6.0 kPa)
- PO$_2$ 44.2 kPa (>10.6 kPa)
- HCO$_3^-$ 15 mEq/L (24–30 mEq/L)
- Base excess −12 mmol/L (+/− 2 mmol/L)

a) What abnormality is shown by the ABG results? *(2 marks)*

b) What additional investigations might help make a diagnosis? *(4 marks)*

The following investigations are performed (normal ranges in brackets):
- Blood glucose 4.1 mmol/L (3.9–5.5 mmol/L)
- Lactate 10 mmol/L (0.6–2.4 mmol/L)
- Blood ketones 1.0 mmol/L (<0.6 mmol/L)
- Na$^+$ 140 mmol/L (135–145 mmol/L)
- K$^+$ 5 mmol/L (3.5–5.3 mmol/L)
- Urea 5.9 mmol/L (2.5–6.7 mmol/L)
- Creatinine 58 µmol/L (70–100 µmol/L)
- Chloride 100 mmol/L (95–105 mmol/L)
- Computed tomography of the head: normal
- Paracetamol/salicylates: not detected
- Blood alcohol 350 mg/dL

c) How do you calculate the anion gap and what is it in this case? *(2 marks)*

d) How does the plasma concentration of albumin affect the anion gap and why? *(2 marks)*

e) Why does acute ethanol intoxication cause a metabolic acidosis? *(4 marks)*

f) The laboratory reports the patient's osmolality as 340 mOsm/kg. How do you calculate the osmolar gap and what is it in this case? *(3 marks)*

g) Other than ethanol intoxication, what other causes are there for an elevated osmolar gap? *(3 marks)*

Answers

a) What abnormality is shown by the ABG results? *(2 marks)*
- Partially compensated ...
- ... metabolic acidosis

b) What additional investigations might help make a diagnosis? *(4 marks)*

  (1 mark per investigation to a maximum of 4)
  - Blood sugar
  - Lactate
  - Blood/urine ketones
  - Urea and electrolytes
  - Chloride
  - Toxicology screen
  - Ethylene glycol levels
  - Blood ethanol levels
  - Computed tomography of the head

c) How do you calculate the anion gap and what is it in this case? *(2 marks)*

- Anion gap = $([Na^+] + [K^+]) - ([Cl^-] + [HCO_3^-])$
- Anion gap = $(140 + 5) - (100 + 15) = 30$ mmol/L

  (In clinical practice, the potassium concentration is occasionally omitted, therefore 25 is also an acceptable answer.)

d) How does the plasma concentration of albumin affect the anion gap and why? *(2 marks)*
- Albumin is the major unmeasured anion and therefore accounts for most of the calculated anion gap
- Every 1 g/L decrease in the albumin concentration will decrease anion gap by 0.25 mmol/L

e) Why does acute ethanol intoxication cause a metabolic acidosis? *(4 marks)*
- Lactate acidosis—ethanol metabolism impairs gluconeogenesis and fatty acid beta-oxidation resulting in increased anaerobic metabolism. Ethanol also impairs the conversion of lactate to pyruvate, reducing lactate clearance
- Alcoholic ketoacidosis—more common in poorly nourished chronic alcoholics a few days after a binge

f) The laboratory reports the patient's osmolality as 340 mOsm/kg. How do you calculate the osmolar gap and what is it in this case? *(3 marks)*
- Osmolar gap = osmolality (measured) − osmolarity (calculated)
- Calculated osmolarity = $2[Na^+] + [glucose] + [urea] = (2 \times 140) + 4.1 + 5.9 = 290$
- Osmolar gap = $340 - 290 = 50$

g) Other than ethanol intoxication, what other causes are there for an elevated osmolar gap? *(3 marks)*

  (1 mark per cause to a maximum of 3)
  - Mannitol
  - Methanol
  - Ethylene glycol
  - Sorbitol
  - Polyethylene glycol
  - Propylene glycol
  - Glycine (TURP syndrome)
  - Hypertriglyceridaemia
  - Hypergammaglobulinaemia

Further reading

Gennari FJ. Current concepts. Serum osmolality. Uses and limitations. *New England Journal of Medicine* 1984;310:102–105.

Kraut JA, Madias NE. Serum anion gap: its uses and limitations in clinical medicine. *Clinical Journal of the American Society of Nephrology* 2007;2:162–174.

FFICM syllabus references 1.1, 2.1, 2.2, 2.5, 2.7, 2.8, 3.1, 3.6, 3.10, 4.8.
CoBaTrICE domains 1, 2, 3.

OSCE 5 station 7—data

Questions

A 74-year-old woman is admitted to the intensive care unit following an emergency Hartmann's procedure for a sigmoid colon perforation with faecal peritonitis. She hadn't eaten anything for 5 days prior to admission and had lost 5 kg of weight over the preceding few weeks. Enteral feeding has been attempted but the nurses are aspirating more than 500 mL from the nasogastric tube every 4 hours.

a) Which drugs could be given to improve gastric emptying? *(2 marks)*

Despite pharmacological management, the nasogastric aspirates do not reduce in volume.

b) What options should be considered? *(2 marks)*

A decision is made to commence total parenteral nutrition (TPN).

c) What are the commonest forms of protein, lipid, and carbohydrate in TPN? *(3 marks)*

d) Complete Table 5.3q with the normal daily requirements for a healthy 70 kg adult *(6 marks)*

Table 5.3q Normal daily requirements for a 70 kg adult

Requirement	Daily amount
Water	____ mL/day
Carbohydrate	____ g/day
Protein	____ g/day
Sodium	____ mmol/day
Potassium	____ mmol/day
Calcium	____ mmol/day

e) The plasma concentrations of which three electrolytes are most commonly affected by refeeding syndrome? *(3 marks)*

f) Other than renal function, trace elements, and electrolytes, which other biochemical tests should be monitored in patients receiving TPN? *(3 marks)*

Answers

a) Which drugs could be given to improve gastric emptying? *(2 marks)*
  - Metoclopramide
  - Erythromycin
b) What options should be considered? *(2 marks)*
  - Nasojejunal feeding
  - Total parenteral nutrition
c) What are the commonest forms of protein, lipid, and carbohydrate in TPN? *(3 marks)*
  - Protein—amino acids
  - Lipid—triglycerides
  - Carbohydrate—glucose
d) Complete Table 5.3a with the normal daily requirements for a healthy 70 kg adult *(6 marks)*

Table 5.3a Normal daily requirements for a 70 kg adult

Requirement	Daily amount
Water	2100 mL/day
Carbohydrate	210–280 g/day
Protein	70–105 g/day
Sodium	70–140 mmol/day
Potassium	50–120 mmol/day
Calcium	5–10 mmol/day

e) The plasma concentrations of which three electrolytes are most commonly affected by refeeding syndrome? *(3 marks)*
  - Phosphate
  - Potassium
  - Magnesium
f) Other than renal function, trace elements, and electrolytes, which other biochemical tests should be monitored in patients receiving TPN? *(3 marks)*

  - Liver function tests
  - Glucose
  - Lipids

Further reading

Kreymann KG, Berger MM, Deutz NEP. ESPEN guidelines on enteral nutrition: intensive care. *Clinical Nutrition* 2006;25:210–223.
Singer P, Berger MM, Van den Berghe G. ESPEN guidelines on parenteral nutrition: intensive care. *Clinical Nutrition* 2009;28:387–400.

FFICM syllabus references 2.2, 3.7, 4.1, 4.8, 4.9, 6.1.
CoBaTrICE domains 3, 4.

OSCE 5 station 8—data

Questions

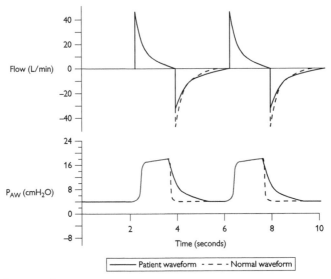

Figure 5.5 Ventilator waveforms

Figure 5.5 shows mandatory pressure-controlled breaths.

a) What problem with the ventilator circuit is shown by these waveforms? *(1 mark)*
b) What are the potential causes of a partial obstruction in the expiratory limb of a ventilator circuit? *(4 marks)*

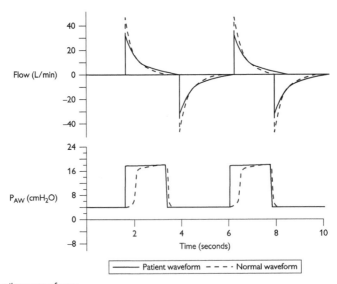

Figure 5.6 Ventilator waveforms

Figure 5.6 also shows mandatory pressure-controlled breaths.

c) What problem is shown on these waveforms? *(1 mark)*
d) What are the equipment-related causes of partial airway obstruction in the ventilated patient? *(3 marks)*

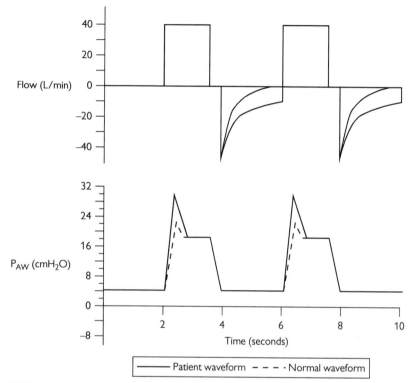

Figure 5.7 flow (L/min), P_{AW} (cmH$_2$O) vs Time (seconds)

Patient waveform ——— Normal waveform – – – ·

Figure 5.7 Ventilator waveforms

Figure 5.7 shows mandatory volume-controlled breaths.

e) What abnormalities are seen on these waveforms? *(2 marks)*
f) How do these waveforms demonstrate that the issue is an increase in resistance rather than a reduction in compliance? *(1 mark)*
g) What measures can be undertaken to allow complete expiration? *(3 marks)*
h) Which ventilator setting changes would increase the expiratory time? *(2 marks)*

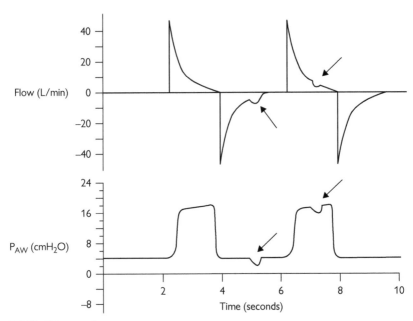

Figure 5.8 Ventilator waveforms

Figure 5.8 shows pressure-controlled breaths.

i) What is happening at the points marked with arrows? *(1 mark)*

j) What are the possible reasons for patient effort not resulting in an assisted breath? *(2 marks)*

Answers

a) What problem with the ventilator circuit is shown by these waveforms? *(1 mark)*
  - Partial obstruction of the expiratory limb
b) What are the potential causes of a partial obstruction in the expiratory limb of a ventilator circuit? *(4 marks)*

  (1 mark per cause to a maximum of 4)
  - Condensed water (rainout)
  - Kinked or compressed tubing
  - Tubing of insufficient diameter (e.g. neonatal tubing used for larger child)
  - Malfunction of the expiratory valve
  - Blockage of the expiratory filter
c) What problem is shown on these waveforms? *(1 mark)*
  - Partial airway obstruction
d) What are the equipment-related causes of partial airway obstruction in the ventilated patient? *(3 marks)*
  - Kinked or compressed endotracheal tube
  - Secretions or blood in the endotracheal tube
  - Blockage of a heat and moisture exchange filter
e) What abnormalities are seen on these waveforms? *(2 marks)*
  - Increased peak airway pressure
  - Incomplete expiration
f) How do these waveforms demonstrate that the issue is an increase in resistance rather than a reduction in compliance? *(1 mark)*
  - The absence of a rise in plateau pressure demonstrates that compliance is unchanged
g) What measures can be undertaken to allow complete expiration? *(3 marks)*
  - Treatment of bronchospasm
  - Reduction of the set tidal volume
  - Increasing the set expiratory time
h) Which ventilator setting changes would increase the expiratory time? *(2 marks)*
  - Decreased respiratory rate (with fixed inspiratory:expiratory ratio)
  - Decreased inspiratory time (with unchanged rate)
i) What is happening at the points marked with arrows? *(1 mark)*
  - The patient is making an inspiratory effort
j) What are the possible reasons for patient effort not resulting in an assisted breath? *(2 marks)*

  - The ventilatory mode does not support assisted ventilation
  - The patient effort is less than the set trigger

Notes

This question builds upon knowledge tested in OSCE 4 station 8.

Further reading

Lei Y. *Medical Ventilator System Basics: A Clinical Guide.* Oxford: Oxford University Press; 2017.

FFICM syllabus references 2.7, 3.8, 4.6.
CoBaTrICE domains 2, 4.

OSCE 5 station 9—data

Questions

A 79-year-old woman was admitted to intensive care 7 days ago following a complicated revision total knee replacement, requiring both cardiovascular and respiratory support. She has a history of atrial fibrillation and a metallic mitral heart valve for which she regularly takes warfarin. You have been asked to assess the patient due to a new swollen calf being detected as well as several necrotic areas of skin over her abdomen. The most recent full blood count is shown as follows (normal ranges in brackets):

- Haemoglobin (Hb) 96 g/L (115–160 g/L)
- Total white cell count (WCC) 15.4 × 10^9/L (4–11 × 10^9/L)
- Neutrophils 13.8 × 10^9/L (2–7.5 × 10^9/L)
- Lymphocytes 1.2 × 10^9/L (1–4.5 × 10^9/L)
- Platelet count 28 × 10^9/L (150–400 × 10^9/L)
- Mean cell volume (MCV) 86 fL (76–96 fL)
- Haematocrit 0.4 L/L (0.37–0.47 L/L)

a) What is the most significant abnormality and what is the most likely cause? *(2 marks)*

b) How can heparin cause thrombocytopenia? *(3 marks)*

c) What are the other common causes of thrombocytopenia in the critically ill? *(3 marks)*

d) What four categories make up the Warkentin (4Ts) heparin-induced thrombocytopenia (HIT) probability score? *(4 marks)*

e) The HIT score demonstrates a high pretest probability for HIT. What action should be taken? *(3 marks)*

f) What laboratory tests are used to confirm the diagnosis of HIT? *(2 marks)*

g) What alternative anticoagulants could be used in patients with HIT? *(3 marks)*

Answers

a) What is the most significant abnormality and what is the most likely cause? *(2 marks)*
- Thrombocytopenia
- Heparin-induced thrombocytopenia

b) How can heparin cause thrombocytopenia? *(3 marks)*
- Heparin binds to platelet factor 4 (PF4), a circulating protein of unclear biological function
- This heparin–PF4 complex is immunogenic, leading to the production of immunoglobulin G (IgG) antibodies (HIT antibodies)
- The heparin–PF4–IgG complex binds to platelets, causing platelet activation and subsequent removal by the reticuloendothelial system

c) What are the other common causes of thrombocytopenia in the critically ill? *(3 marks)*

(1 mark per cause to a maximum of 3)
- Dilution—unbalanced transfusion
- Consumption—sepsis, bleeding, disseminated intravascular coagulation, extracorporeal circuits and devices, trauma, thrombotic thrombocytopenic purpura, idiopathic thrombocytopenic purpura
- Reduced production—hepatic failure, sepsis, drug induced, critical illness marrow suppression
- Destruction—autoimmune disease, drug induced
- Sequestration—hypersplenism, hypothermia

d) What four clinical features make up the Warkentin (4Ts) HIT probability score? *(4 marks)*
- Magnitude of *T*hrombocytopenia
- *T*iming (of thrombocytopenia or thrombosis or other clinical sequelae, in relation to the initiation of a course of heparin)
- The presence of *T*hrombosis (or other clinical sequelae)
- The presence of o*T*her potential non-HIT explanations for thrombocytopenia or clinical events observed

e) The HIT score demonstrates a high pretest probability for HIT. What action should be taken? *(3 marks)*
- An alternative anticoagulant should be initiated
- Heparin should be withdrawn
- The diagnosis should be confirmed

f) What laboratory tests are used to confirm the diagnosis of HIT? *(2 marks)*
- Immunoassays detect the presence of the presence of HIT antibodies in the plasma
- Functional platelet assays measure platelet activity in the presence of heparin, donated platelets, and the patient's own plasma

g) What alternative anticoagulants could be used in patients with HIT? *(3 marks)*

(1 mark per anticoagulant to a maximum of 3)
- Bivalirudin
- Argatroban
- Danaparoid
- Fondaparinux

Further reading

Linkins LA. Clinical Review. Heparin induced thrombocytopenia. *BMJ* 2015;350:g7566.

FFICM syllabus references 1.1, 2.2, 2.8, 3.1, 4.1, 6.1, 11.4, 11.7.
CoBaTrICE domains 2,3,6.

OSCE 5 station 10—data

Questions

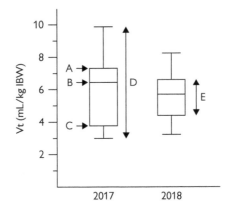

Figure 5.9 Results

Your colleagues have completed the second cycle of an audit of tidal volumes. They have presented the data as shown in Figure 5.9.

a) What type of chart is shown in Figure 5.9? *(1 mark)*
b) What do labels A–E signify? *(5 marks)*
c) Why is the median used as the descriptor of central tendency rather than the mean? *(1 mark)*
d) How does the position of the median line within the box indicate the skew of data? *(2 marks)*

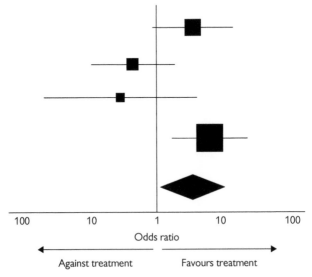

Figure 5.10 Results

The chart shown in Figure 5.10 is from the results section of a meta-analysis.

e) What type of chart is shown in Figure 5.10? *(1 mark)*

f) How many studies were included in this meta-analysis? *(1 mark)*

g) What do the horizontal lines protruding from each square represent? *(1 mark)*

h) What does the horizontal position of each square represent? *(1 mark)*

i) What does the size of the square represent? *(1 mark)*

j) What does the width of the diamond represent? *(1 mark)*

k) How do you know that this meta-analysis reported a statistically significant outcome? *(1 mark)*

l) By what name is the y-axis known in a forest plot? *(1 mark)*

m) Why might relevant evidence not be included in a meta-analysis? *(2 marks)*

n) What name is given to the bias produced by the non-publication of negative studies? *(1 mark)*

Answers

a) What type of chart is shown in Figure 5.9? *(1 mark)*
- A box (and) whisker chart

b) What do labels A–E signify? *(5 marks)*

A 75th centile

B median

C 25th centile

D range

E interquartile range

c) Why is the median used as the descriptor of central tendency rather than the mean? *(1 mark)*
- The mean is used with parametric data; this data is non-parametric

d) How does the position of the median line within the box indicate the skew of data? *(2 marks)*
- If the median line is not central in the box the data is skewed
- If the line is above the midpoint the data is positively skewed and vice versa

e) What type of chart is shown in Figure 5.10? *(1 mark)*
- A forest plot

f) How many studies were included in this meta-analysis? *(1 mark)*
- Four

g) What do the horizontal lines protruding from each square represent? *(1 mark)*
- The stated confidence interval of the study

h) What does the horizontal position of each square represent? *(1 mark)*
- The odds ratio found in each original study

i) What does the size of the square represent? *(1 mark)*
- The weight (power) given to each study in the meta-analysis

j) What does the width of the diamond represent? *(1 mark)*
- The stated confidence interval for the combined odds ratio

k) How do you know that this meta-analysis reported a statistically significant outcome? *(1 mark)*
- The diamond does not cross the y-axis

l) By what name is the y-axis known in a forest plot? *(1 mark)*
- The line of no effect

m) Why might relevant evidence not be included in a meta-analysis? *(2 marks)*

(1 mark per reason to a maximum of 2)
- The evidence may not have been published
- The study may be inaccessible or written in a foreign language
- Incomplete literature search

n) What name is given to the bias produced by the non-publication of negative studies? *(1 mark)*
- Publication bias

Notes

This is a 'know it or you don't' question, but it includes all you could ever really be asked about box–whisker and forest plots.

Further reading

Cochrane UK. How to read a forest plot? Available at: http://uk.cochrane.org/news/how-read-forest-plot [accessed 21 May 2018].

FFICM syllabus references 12.13, 12.15.
CoBaTrICE domain 11.

OSCE 5 station 11—data

Questions

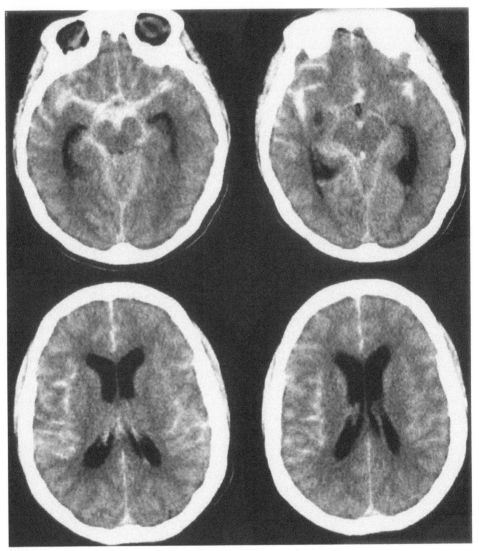

Figure 5.11 CT head
Reproduced from *Oxford Textbook of Stroke and Cardiovascular Disease*, Norrving B, Figure 6.18. © 2014 Oxford University Press.
Reproduced with permission of the Licensor through PLSclear

Look at the computed tomography (CT) scan in Figure 5.11.

a) What is the diagnosis? *(1 mark)*
b) What scoring systems are used to grade the severity of aneurysmal subarachnoid haemorrhage? *(3 marks)*
c) What are the systemic complications of subarachnoid haemorrhage *(5 marks)*

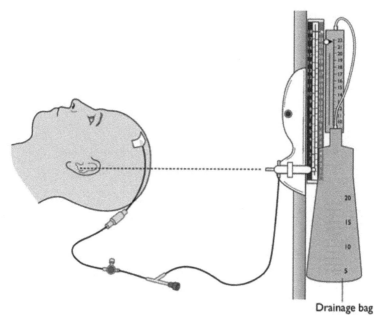

Drainage bag

Figure 5.12 Medical device

Reproduced from *Oxford Handbook of Operative Surgery, Third Edition*, Agarwal A, Borley B, and Mclatchie G, Figure 13.6. © 2017 Oxford University Press. Reproduced with permission of the Licensor through PLSclear

Look at Figure 5.12.

d) What is this device? *(1 mark)*

e) Why might an external ventricular drain be useful in acute subarachnoid haemorrhage? *(3 marks)*

f) What definitive treatment options are available for aneurysmal subarachnoid haemorrhage? *(2 marks)*

g) What does the International Subarachnoid Aneurysm Trial (ISAT) tell us about the efficacy of endovascular coiling? *(3 marks)*

h) What features of an aneurysm make neurosurgical clipping preferable to coiling? *(2 marks)*

Answers

a) What is the diagnosis? *(1 mark)*
- Subarachnoid haemorrhage

b) What scoring systems are used to grade the severity of aneurysmal subarachnoid haemorrhage? *(3 marks)*

(1 mark per scoring system to a maximum of 3)
- Clinical:
  - Glasgow Coma Score
  - Prognosis on Admission of Aneurysmal Subarachnoid Haemorrhage (PAASH) score
  - World Federation of Neurosurgeons (WFNS) grading
  - Hunt and Hess score
- Radiological:
  - Fischer and modified Fischer grading
  - Claassen CT rating scale
- Hybrid of clinical and radiological scores:
  - Vasograde score

c) What are the systemic complications of subarachnoid haemorrhage *(5 marks)*

(1 mark per complication to a maximum of 5)
- Cardiac—myocardial injury, dysrhythmias, global and regional wall motion abnormalities including takotsubo cardiomyopathy
- Respiratory—neurogenic pulmonary oedema, aspiration pneumonitis
- Endocrine—hyperglycaemia, pyrexia, hyponatraemia (cerebral salt-wasting syndrome, syndrome of inappropriate antidiuretic hormone)
- Gastrointestinal—stress ulceration
- Haematological—venous thromboembolism

d) What is this device? *(1 mark)*
- External ventricular drain

e) Why might an external ventricular drain be useful in acute subarachnoid haemorrhage? *(3 marks)*
- Acute hydrocephalus occurs in approximately 20% of patients with subarachnoid haemorrhage
- An external ventricular device can be used to drain cerebrospinal fluid (reducing intracranial hypertension)
- … and as a gold standard intracranial pressure monitoring device

f) What definitive treatment options are available for aneurysmal subarachnoid haemorrhage? *(2 marks)*
- Endovascular coiling
- Neurosurgical clipping

g) What does the International Subarachnoid Aneurysm Trial (ISAT) tell us about the efficacy of endovascular coiling? *(3 marks)*

(1 mark per finding to a maximum of 3)
When compared with clipping, coiling was associated with:
- Reduction in death or severe neurological deficit at 1 year (7.4% absolute risk reduction)
- Survival benefit sustained at 7 years
- Lower rate of post-procedure epilepsy and cognitive decline
- Increased post treatment rebleeding in the first year

h) What features of an aneurysm make neurosurgical clipping preferable to coiling? *(2 marks)*
- Middle cerebral artery territory aneurysm
- Aneurysm with a wide neck or with close association to arterial tributaries

Further reading

D'Oliviera Manoel A, Turkel-Parrella D, Duggal A, Murphy A, McCredie V, Marotta T. Managing aneurysmal sub-arachnoid haemorrhage: it takes a team. *Cleveland Clinic Journal of Medicine* 2015;82:177–192.

Steiner T, Juvela S, Unterberg A, Jung C, Forsting M, Rinkel G. European Stroke Organisation guidelines for the management of intracranial aneurysms and subarachnoid haemorrhage. *Cerebrovascular Diseases* 2013;35:93–112.

FFICM syllabus references 2.6, 3.1, 3.6, 11.7.
CoBaTrICE domains 2, 3, 4.

OSCE 5 station 12—equipment

Questions

a) What three elements are required for a fire to start? *(3 marks)*

b) What is the most common type of fire in the intensive care unit? *(1 mark)*

c) How might the spread of a fire on the intensive care unit be contained? *(4 marks)*

d) What types of fire extinguisher should *not* be used on an electrical fire? *(2 marks)*

e) What precautions should be taken when storing oxygen cylinders to reduce the risk of fire? *(4 marks)*

f) What terms are used to describe the types of patient evacuation from hospitals? *(3 marks)*

g) In what order should patients be evacuated when there is a fire in the intensive care unit? *(2 marks)*

A mechanically ventilated patient is being evacuated from the intensive care unit and is receiving 100% oxygen with a minute volume of 9 L per minute from a size E cylinder. The patient is attached to a portable ventilator which has a driving gas (oxygen) consumption of 1 L per minute.

h) Assuming the cylinder was full, how many minutes of oxygen supply are available before the cylinder is empty? *(1 mark)*

Answers

a) What three elements are required for a fire to start? *(3 marks)*
- Heat
- Fuel
- Oxygen

b) What is the most common type of fire in the intensive care unit? *(1 mark)*
- Electrical fire

c) How might the spread of a fire on the intensive care unit be contained? *(4 marks)*
- Turning off oxygen outlets
- Closing windows and doors
- Incorporating fire barrier walls and doors in building design
- Extinguishing the fire

d) What types of fire extinguisher should *not* be used on an electrical fire? *(2 marks)*
- Water extinguishers
- Foam extinguishers

e) What precautions should be taken when storing oxygen cylinders to reduce the risk of fire? *(4 marks)*

(1 mark per precaution to a maximum of 4)
- Handling oxygen cylinders carefully
- Keeping cylinders chained or clamped to prevent them from falling over
- Storing oxygen cylinders in a well-dedicated storage area
- Storing oxygen cylinders away from combustible materials
- Storing oxygen cylinders in a well-ventilated area
- Storing the minimum number of cylinders as possible
- Returning empty cylinders to the supplier as soon as possible
- Treating empty cylinders with the same caution full cylinders

f) What terms are used to describe the types of patient evacuation from hospitals? *(3 marks)*
- Horizontal evacuation (through a fire door to an adjacent area)
- Vertical evacuation (to a lower floor)
- External evacuation (out of the building)

g) In what order should patients should be evacuated when there is a fire in the intensive care unit? *(2 marks)*
- Patients in the immediate vicinity of the fire (where safe to do so) …
- … then the most stable patients before unstable patients

h) Assuming the cylinder was full, how many minutes of oxygen supply are available before the cylinder is empty? *(1 mark)*
- 68 minutes

(Size E oxygen cylinder supplies 680 L of oxygen and required volume = 10 L per minute.)

Further reading

Kelly FE, Hardy R, Cook TM, Nolan JP, Craft T, Osborn M, et al. Managing the aftermath of a fire on intensive care caused by an oxygen cylinder. *Journal of the Intensive Care Society* 2014;15:283–287.

Kelly FE, Hardy R, Hall EA, McDonald J, Turner M, Rivers J, et al. Fire on an intensive care unit caused by an oxygen cylinder. *Anaesthesia* 2013;68:102–104.

London Critical Care Network. Principles of evacuation and shelter for critical care. Available at: https://www.londonccn.nhs.uk [accessed 2 May 2019].

FFICM syllabus references 5.1, 10.1, 11.3, 11.8, 12.11.
CoBaTrICE domains 11, 12.

OSCE 5 station 13—equipment

Questions

a) With relevance to pulse oximetry, what is Lambert's law *(1 mark)*
b) With relevance to pulse oximetry, what are isosbestic points, and at what wavelengths do they occur? *(2 marks)*
c) What are the wavelengths of the two light sources in a pulse oximeter? *(2 marks)*

A patient is brought to the emergency department from a nightclub. He was found collapsed, having previously been seen with a small brown bottle. An initial assessment shows:

- Cyanosis
- SpO_2 85%
- Heart rate of 120 beats per minute
- Respiratory rate of 16 breaths per minute
- Methaemoglobin concentration of 25%

d) What is the likely cause of this presentation? *(1 mark)*
e) Why is the patient cyanosed? *(2 marks)*
f) Other than the presence of methaemoglobin, what other factors increase the affinity of haemoglobin for oxygen? *(4 marks)*
g) Why is the pulse oximeter recording a saturation of 85%? *(1 mark)*
h) Other than the presence of abnormal haemoglobins or dyes, in what other situations might pulse oximetry be inaccurate? *(5 marks)*
i) What treatment should be given to a patient who has ingested a volatile nitrite? *(2 marks)*

Answers

a) With relevance to pulse oximetry, what is Lambert's law *(1 mark)*
  - The absorption of radiation by a substance is directly proportional to the thickness of the absorbing layer

b) With relevance to pulse oximetry, what are isosbestic points, and at what wavelengths do they occur? *(2 marks)*
  - Isosbestic points are wavelengths at which the absorption of light is equal for oxyhaemoglobin and deoxyhaemoglobin
  - 590 nm and 805 nm

c) What are the wavelengths of the two light sources in a pulse oximeter? *(2 marks)*
  - 660 nm
  - 940 nm

d) What is the likely cause of this presentation? *(1 mark)*
  - Ingestion of a volatile nitrite (e.g. amyl nitrite)

e) Why is the patient cyanosed? *(2 marks)*
  - Nitrites oxidize the haem molecule from a ferrous (Fe^{2+}) to a ferric (Fe^{3+}) state, forming methaemoglobin, which in turn reduces the oxygen-carrying capacity of the blood
  - In addition, the presence of methaemoglobin changes the shape of the haemoglobin molecule. This change in shape increases the affinity of haemoglobin for oxygen, reducing the off-loading of oxygen to the tissues

f) Other than the presence of methaemoglobin, what other factors increase the affinity of haemoglobin for oxygen? *(4 marks)*
  - Increased pH
  - Reduced temperature
  - Reduced PCO_2
  - Reduced levels of 2,3-bisphosphoglycerate (2,3-BPG)

g) Why is the pulse oximeter recording a saturation of 85%? *(1 mark)*
  - Methaemoglobin absorbs red and infrared light at the wavelengths of 660 nm and 940 nm. The measured absorbance is like that seen with an oxygen saturation of 85% in the absence of methaemoglobin

h) Other than the presence of abnormal haemoglobins or dyes, in what other situations might pulse oximetry be inaccurate? *(5 marks)*
  - Reduced tissue perfusion (e.g. shock)
  - Venous pulsation (e.g. tricuspid regurgitation)
  - Motion artefact (e.g. shivering)
  - Physical barriers (e.g. nail polish)
  - Electrical interference (e.g. use of diathermy)

i) What treatment should be given to a patient who has ingested a volatile nitrite? *(2 marks)*
  - Oxygen
  - Methylthioninium chloride (methylene blue) 1–2 mg/kg intravenously acts as a reducing agent, reducing the amount of methaemoglobin present. The dose can be repeated as necessary

Notes

It's important to remember that the syllabus (and therefore potentially the exam) contains a huge amount of basic science.

Further reading

Hunter L, Gordge L, Dargan Pl, Wood DM. Methaemoglobinaemia associated with the use of cocaine and volatile nitrites as recreational drugs: a review. *British Journal of Clinical Pharmacology* 2011;72:18–26.

Ralston AC, Webb RK, Runciman WB. Potential errors in pulse oximetry III: effects of interference, dyes, dyshaemoglobins and other pigments. *Anaesthesia* 1991;46:291–295.

FFICM syllabus references 1.1, 2.1, 2.2, 2.7, 2.8, 3.10, 4.1.
CoBaTrICE domains 1, 2.

OSCE 6

OSCE 6 station 1—professionalism

Questions

a) What could be achieved by conducting a case conference? *(4 marks)*

You are caring for a patient on the intensive care unit who is severely functionally impaired (nursing home resident, bed bound, unable to communicate, and dependent on others for all activities of daily living) due a traumatic head injury 20 years ago. The patient has been ventilated after an episode of aspiration pneumonia and has made little progress in weaning from the ventilator. You are considering whether a tracheostomy would be in her best interests so decide to organize a case conference.

b) Who do you think should be invited to take part in the case conference? *(6 marks)*
c) The departmental secretary agrees to attend, but he would like to know what he should document? *(4 marks)*
d) He would also like to know where the record of the case conference should be held? *(1 mark)*

During the case conference, a conflict occurs between the family and the respiratory physician.

e) What strategies could you use to resolve the conflict? *(5 marks)*

Answers

a) What could be achieved by conducting a case conference? *(4 marks)*

(1 mark per goal to a maximum of 4)
- Determining best interests
- Defining treatment aims and goals
- Reviewing progress with treatment
- Identifying and overcoming barriers
- Defining roles and responsibilities
- Resolving conflict

b) Who do you think should be invited to take part in the case conference? *(6 marks)*

(1 mark per individual to a maximum of 6)
- Patient advocate—e.g. family, attorney, independent mental capacity advocate (IMCA), friend, etc.
- Primary healthcare providers—e.g. nursing home staff, general practitioner, community therapists
- Secondary healthcare specialists—e.g. critical care, palliative care, respiratory medicine, neurorehabilitation
- Secondary healthcare professionals—e.g. physiotherapists, critical care nursing staff
- Outside and supporting agencies—e.g. social services, charity case workers, chaplaincy
- Secretarial staff

c) The departmental secretary agrees to attend, but he would like to know what he should document? *(4 marks)*
- Consent for the conference to take place (provided by the healthcare team or attorney if the patient does not have capacity)
- The time and date of the meeting
- A register of attendees
- A summary of the discussion and any action plan

d) He would also like to know where the record of the case conference should be held? *(1 mark)*
- Within the patient record

e) What strategies could you use to resolve the conflict? *(5 marks)*

(1 mark per strategy to a maximum of 5)
- Acknowledge that a conflict is occurring—one party may be unaware
- Acknowledge both viewpoints as having equal value
- Ensure each party can explain their point of view fully including the reasons for holding it
- Try to identify the source of the conflict—'what is the real issue'?
- Ensure the discussion concerns the issue, not the individuals involved
- Establish any facts and areas of common ground
- State that resolution may require later discussion

Notes

Organizing a case conference is a syllabus item but there's not much that could be asked that isn't part of this question!

FFICM syllabus references 11.5, 12.2, 12.3, 12.4, 12.7, 12.8.
CoBaTrICE domain 12.

OSCE 6 station 2—resuscitation

Questions

You have been called to the emergency department to see an 8-year-old child (weight 30 kg) who is known to have a sesame allergy and has developed tongue swelling after eating a sandwich.

The parents tell you that their adrenaline autoinjector was past its expiry date, and that they think the tongue swelling is getting worse. No medications have been given.

a) What specific clinical findings would you look for in a child with anaphylaxis? *(4 marks)*
b) What else would you be doing while assessing the child? *(5 marks)*

On your assessment you find:

A—stridor, obviously swollen tongue
B—no wheeze, respiratory rate 32 breaths per minute, saturations 94% on room air
C—heart rate 140 beats per minute, blood pressure 90/45 mmHg, capillary refill is 4 seconds
D—alert but tearful, temperature 39.6°C
E—widespread urticarial rash

c) What therapies (and at what dose) are you going to give the child? *(10 marks)*
d) What investigation should be performed to confirm the diagnosis? *(1 mark)*

Answers

a) What specific clinical findings would you look for in a child with anaphylaxis? *(4 marks)*
- Signs of upper airway obstruction, e.g. oral swelling, stridor, hoarse voice
- Signs of bronchospasm, e.g. hypoxia, tachypnoea, wheeze, increased work of breathing
- Signs of shock, e.g. tachycardia, hypotension, pallor, prolonged capillary refill time, altered consciousness
- Skin changes, e.g. conjunctival injection, urticaria, erythema, angio-oedema

b) What else would you be doing while assessing the child? *(5 marks)*
- Applying monitoring
- Applying oxygen
- Calling for help
- Asking for medications to be prepared
- Siting intravenous (IV) access

c) What therapies (and at what dose) are you going to give the child? *(10 marks)*

(1 mark per drug and 1 mark per correct dose)
- Intramuscular (IM) adrenaline   10 mcg/kg = 300 mcg = 0.3 mL 1:1000
- Nebulized adrenaline   5 mL of 1:1000
- IV fluid bolus   20 mL/kg = 600 mL of crystalloid
- IM/slow IV hydrocortisone   100 mg
- IM/slow IV chlorphenamine   5 mg

(No marks for salbutamol as the child does not have wheeze.)

d) What investigation should be performed to confirm the diagnosis? *(1 mark)*
- Mast cell tryptase

Notes

The temptation in this scenario would be to focus on the airway compromise and to forget to assess and treat the whole patient. There will not be any scenarios where the first marks available are for inducing anaesthesia, so if that is your first action marks will be lost.

While IV adrenaline is a treatment option, the marks in this question are for the more strongly recommended IM route.

Further reading

Resuscitation Council (UK). Emergency treatment of anaphylactic reaction—guidelines. 2008. Available at: https:// www.resus.org.uk/anaphylaxis/emergency-treatment-of-anaphylactic-reactions [accessed 11 October 2018].

FFICM syllabus references 2.1, 2.2, 4.1, 4.4, 9.1.
CoBaTrICE domains 9.

OSCE 6 station 3—data

Questions

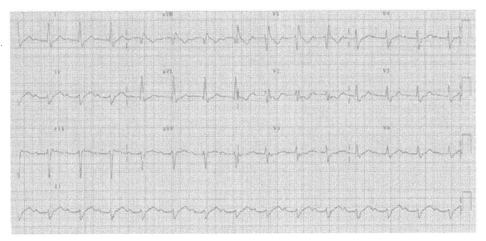

Figure 6.1 Electrocardiogram (ECG)

Reproduced from *Emergencies in Cardiology, Second Edition*, Myerson SG et al., Figure 21.23. © 2009 Oxford University Press. Reproduced with permission of the Licensor through PLSclear

A 75-year-old patient with ischaemic heart disease has been admitted to hospital with recurrent syncopal episodes. An echocardiograph shows moderate biventricular dysfunction and cardiac angiography demonstrates a chronically occluded right coronary artery with diffuse coronary disease.

Drug history—bisoprolol, ramipril, spironolactone and furosemide.

Look at Figure 6.1.

a) What abnormalities are present on this electrocardiogram (ECG)? *(4 marks)*

b) What are the likely causes of trifascicular block in this patient? *(3 marks)*

A temporary pacing wire is inserted.

c) How could you describe temporary pacing wires using the first three positions of the British Pacing and Electrophysiology Group generic pacemaker code? *(2 marks)*

d) When present, what is the significance of the fourth and fifth letter of the generic pacemaker code? *(2 marks)*

e) With reference to pacemaker functionality, what is rate modulation? *(1 mark)*

f) What actions should be taken when defibrillating a patient with a permanent pacemaker? *(2 marks)*

g) How would you disable the defibrillation function of an implantable cardioverter defibrillator (ICD) in an emergency? *(2 marks)*

A patient has a biventricular pacemaker with a defibrillator function. End of life care has been discussed and agreed.

h) What specific steps need to be taken regarding the device? *(4 marks)*

Answers

a) What abnormalities are present on this electrocardiogram (ECG)? *(4 marks)*
  - First-degree atrioventricular block
  - Left axis deviation
  - Right bundle branch block
  - Trifascicular block

b) What are the likely causes of trifascicular block in this patient? *(3 marks)*
  - Ischaemic heart disease
  - Biventricular dysfunction
  - Medication effects—beta blockers, calcium channel blockers, or electrolyte abnormalities due to diuretic use

c) How could you describe temporary pacing wires using the first three positions of the British Pacing and Electrophysiology Group generic pacemaker code? *(2 marks)*
  - VVI for demand pacing (paced ventricle, sensed ventricle, inhibited if native activity sensed) *or*
  - VOO for fixed asynchronous pacing (paced ventricle, no sensing)

d) When present, what is the significance of the fourth and fifth positions of the generic pacemaker code? *(2 marks)*
  - Fourth position—R if rate modulation is present, O if not
  - Fifth position—denotes if the pacemaker is pacing at more than one site in the atrium (A), ventricle (V), or both (D). If not present, O is used

e) With reference to pacemaker functionality, what is rate modulation? *(1 mark)*
  - The ability of the pacemaker to alter the rate based on physiological demand

f) What actions should be taken when defibrillating a patient with a permanent pacemaker? *(2 marks)*
  - The defibrillator pads should be placed as far from the pacing box as possible
  - The pacemaker must be checked as soon as possible post defibrillation to check the pacemaker settings and functionality

g) How would you disable the defibrillation function of an implantable cardioverter defibrillator (ICD) in an emergency? *(2 marks)*
  - Deactivation of the rhythm detection and defibrillation functions can be performed by placing a ring magnet over the pacemaker box
  - The magnet must remain over the pacemaker box to ensure the defibrillator function remains deactivated

h) What specific steps need to be taken regarding the device? *(4 marks)*
  - Early planning and shared decision-making are paramount (discussions surrounding deactivation should take place at the time of consent for the device)
  - Deactivation of ICD function should be performed by the cardiac physiologist in non-emergent situations or by using a ring magnet in an emergency, to avoid shock delivery at the end of life
  - It may be desirable to keep certain functions active, e.g.:
    * In pacemaker dependency (due to insufficient native rhythm), death would be immediate on disabling the pacemaker
    * In severe heart failure, the cardiac resynchronization function of the pacemaker may be kept active for symptom control while the defibrillator function is deactivated

Further reading

Pitcher D, Soar J, Hogg K, Linker N, Chapman S, et al. Cardiovascular implanted electronic devices in people towards the end of life, during cardiopulmonary resuscitation and after death: Guidance from the Resuscitation Council (UK), British Cardiovascular Society and National Council for Palliative Care. *Heart* 2016;102:A1–A17.

FFICM syllabus references 2.2, 2.3, 3.1, 3.2, 3.3, 4.5, 5.11, 5.12, 7.1, 8.1, 8.3, 12.12.
CoBaTrICE domains 1, 2, 3, 4, 8.

OSCE 6 station 4—data

Questions

A 54-year-old man with a 20-year history of alcohol misuse has been admitted to hospital with a 3-week history of increasing shortness of breath. He has clinical and radiological signs of pulmonary oedema. He denies chest pain and has no previous cardiac history.

His blood pressure is 102/42 mmHg, heart rate is 115 beats per minute, and his SpO_2 is 92% in air.

An electrocardiogram shows atrial fibrillation (rate 115 beats per minute) with broad QRS complexes.

a) What features on a chest X-ray suggest interstitial pulmonary oedema? *(3 marks)*

b) What is the NHS definition of alcohol misuse? *(1 mark)*

c) What are the different types of cardiomyopathy? *(5 marks)*

d) How is dilated cardiomyopathy defined? *(2 marks)*

e) Which autoimmune diseases can cause dilated cardiomyopathy? *(3 marks)*

f) What first-line pharmacological therapies should be recommended to this patient once the acute pulmonary oedema has been adequately treated? *(5 marks)*

g) Which vitamin deficiency is a rare cause of alcohol-related heart failure? *(1 mark)*

Answers

a) What features on a chest X-ray suggest interstitial pulmonary oedema? *(3 marks)*
  - Peribronchial cuffing
  - Septal lines (Kerley lines)
  - Thickening of interlobar fissures

b) What is the NHS definition of alcohol misuse? *(1 mark)*

  - Regularly (most weeks) drinking >14 units of alcohol per week

c) What are the different types of cardiomyopathy? *(5 marks)*
  - Dilated
  - Restrictive
  - Hypertrophic
  - Arrhythmogenic right ventricular
  - Unclassified

d) How is dilated cardiomyopathy defined? *(2 marks)*

  - Left ventricular dilatation and left ventricular systolic dysfunction
  - … in the absence of pressure/volume overload or significant ischaemic impairment

e) Which autoimmune diseases can cause dilated cardiomyopathy? *(3 marks)*

  (1 mark per disease to a maximum of 3)
  - Granulomatosis with polyangiitis
  - Sarcoidosis
  - Amyloidosis
  - Lupus
  - Polyarteritis nodosa

f) What first-line pharmacological therapies should be recommended to this patient once the acute pulmonary oedema has been adequately treated? *(5 marks)*
  - Angiotensin-converting enzyme inhibitor
  - Beta blocker
  - Diuretics
  - Rate/rhythm control
  - Consideration of anticoagulation

g) Which vitamin deficiency is a rare cause of alcohol-related heart failure? *(1 mark)*
  - Thiamine deficiency (wet beriberi)

Further reading

National Institute for Health and Care Excellence (NICE). Acute heart failure: diagnosis and management: NICE Guideline [NG187]. 2014. Available at: https://www.nice.org.uk/guidance/ng187 [accessed 15 May 2019].

National Institute for Health and Care Excellence (NICE). Chronic heart failure in adults: diagnosis and management: NICE Guideline [NG106]. 2018. Available at: https://www.nice.org.uk/guidance/ng106 [accessed 15 May 2019].

FFICM syllabus references 1.1, 2.2, 2.3, 2.6, 2.8, 3.1, 3.2, 3.3, 4.1, 12.4.
CoBaTrICE domains 1, 2, 3.

OSCE 6 station 5—data

Questions

A 30-year-old woman who is 36 weeks pregnant has been admitted to the antenatal ward with right upper quadrant pain, nausea, vomiting, and malaise. Her pregnancy has been uncomplicated with no concerns during her routine antenatal screening and care. She has no significant past medical history and no history of drug or alcohol misuse.

Examination:

A—patent

B—respiratory rate 30 breaths per minute, saturations 96% on room air

C—heart rate 118 beats per minute, blood pressure 142/62 mmHg

D—Glasgow Coma Scale score 14 (E4, V4, M6)

E—temperature 37.0°C. No signs of chronic liver disease

Investigations (normal ranges in brackets):

- Urinalysis dipstick—protein 2+, white cells, blood, and nitrites negative
- Haemoglobin 108 g/L (115–160 g/L), white cell count 15×10^9/L (4–11 10^9/L), platelets 100×10^9/L (150–400 10^9/L)
- Prothrombin time 22 seconds (10–14 seconds), activated partial thromboplastin time 50 seconds (35–45 seconds)
- Sodium 138 mmol/L (135–145 mmol/L), potassium 4 mmol/L (3.4–5.3 mmol/L)
- Urea 8 mmol/L (2.5–6.7 mmol/L), creatinine 150 µmol/L (70–100 µmol/L)
- Alkaline phosphatase (ALP) 128 U/L (30–130 U/L), bilirubin 178 µmol/L (3–17 µmol/L), alanine aminotransferase (ALT) 480 IU/L (5–35 IU/L), gamma-glutamyl transferase (GGT) 380 IU/L (7–33 IU/L)
- Glucose 3 mmol/L (3.5–5.5)
- C-reactive protein, bile acids, and amylase—within normal limits
- Paracetamol—undetectable

Imaging:

- Abdominal ultrasound—normal renal and biliary architecture, normal hepatic and portal blood flow, and absence of hepatic infarction, haematoma, or rupture
- Fetal scan—normal growth and nil abnormalities

a) What are the pregnancy-specific differential diagnoses? *(3 marks)*
b) What are the diagnostic criteria for pre-eclampsia? *(6 marks)*
c) What does the acronym HELLP stand for? *(1 mark)*
d) What investigations would demonstrate haemolysis and therefore support a diagnosis of HELLP? *(4 marks)*
e) What pattern of laboratory findings would you expect in a patient who has developed acute fatty liver disease (AFLD) of pregnancy? *(4 marks)*
f) What is the definitive management of AFLD of pregnancy? *(1 mark)*
g) Following delivery, what is the natural history of AFLD? *(1 mark)*

Answers

a) What are the pregnancy-specific differential diagnoses? *(3 marks)*
   - HELLP
   - Acute fatty liver of pregnancy
   - Pre-eclampsia

b) What are the diagnostic criteria for pre-eclampsia? *(6 marks)*
   - New onset, persistent hypertension (two readings, at least 4 hours apart) …
   - … after 20 weeks' gestation
   - … defined as systolic blood pressure >139 mmHg or diastolic blood pressure >89 mmHg
   - … with one or more of the following features:
     - Proteinuria
     - Systemic involvement
     - Uteroplacental dysfunction/fetal growth restriction

c) What does the acronym HELLP stand for? *(1 mark)*
   - Haemolysis, elevated liver enzymes, and low platelets

d) What investigations would demonstrate haemolysis and therefore support a diagnosis of HELLP? *(4 marks)*
   - Microangiopathic haemolysis on a blood film with fragmented cells, i.e. schistocytes or helmet cells
   - Raised lactate dehydrogenase
   - Raised indirect bilirubin
   - Low serum haptoglobin concentration

e) What pattern of laboratory findings would you expect in a patient who has developed acute fatty liver disease (AFLD) of pregnancy? *(4 marks)*

   (1 mark for each finding to a maximum of 4)
   - Encephalopathy with elevated ammonia
   - Hypoglycaemia
   - Severe derangement of aminotransferases (3–15 × the upper normal limit for pregnancy)
   - Elevated bilirubin (4–15 × the upper normal limit for pregnancy)
   - Disseminated intravascular coagulation or severe coagulopathy
   - Elevated creatinine
   - Elevated uric acid
   - Leucocytosis

f) What is the definitive management for AFLD of pregnancy? *(1 mark)*
   - Delivery of the fetus irrespective of gestational age and multidisciplinary supportive care for the mother

g) Following delivery, what is the typical history of AFLD? *(1 mark)*
   - Resolution of liver and renal dysfunction within 7–10 days

Further reading

Westbrook RH, Dusheiko G, Williamson C. Pregnancy and liver disease. *Journal of Hepatology* 2016;64:933–945.

FFICM syllabus references 2.2, 2.8, 3.5.
CoBaTrICE domains 2, 3.

OSCE 6 station 6—data

Questions

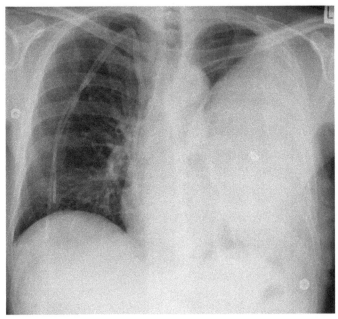

Figure 6.2 Chest X-ray

Reproduced from *Thoracic Imaging*, Desai SR *et al.*, Figure 10.3. © 2012 Oxford University Press. Reproduced with permission of the Licensor through PLSclear

A 62-year-old woman has been admitted to the emergency department with a 3-day history of fever, rigors, and breathlessness. She is currently undergoing chemotherapy for breast cancer. Her respiratory rate is 32 breaths per minute and oxygen saturations are 94% on 8 L per minute of oxygen.

Look at Figure 6.2.

a) What are the main findings on this chest X-ray? *(2 marks)*

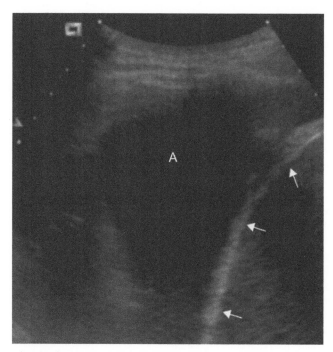

Figure 6.3 Chest ultrasound

Reproduced from *Thoracic Imaging*, Desai SR *et al.*, Figure 10.8a. © 2012 Oxford University Press. Reproduced with permission of the Licensor through PLSclear

Look at Figure 6.3.

b) What is marked by the arrows and area A? *(2 marks)*

c) What investigation should be performed to evaluate the pleural effusion? *(1 mark)*

d) What tests are commonly performed on aspirated pleural fluid? *(7 marks)*

e) What is the purpose of Light's criteria? *(1 mark)*

f) Which biochemical findings make an exudate more likely according to Light's criteria? *(3 marks)*

g) How can the pleural fluid albumin concentration be useful in deciding if an exudate is likely? *(1 mark)*

The pH of the fluid is 7.02 (normal range: 7.35–7.45) and glucose is half of serum level.

h) What are the two most likely causes of this effusion? *(2 marks)*

i) What would be the next therapeutic intervention? *(1 marks)*

Answers

a) What are the main findings on this chest X-ray? *(2 marks)*
   - Large left-sided pleural effusion
   - Hickman line

b) What is marked by the arrows and area A? *(2 marks)*
   - Arrows—diaphragm
   - Area A—pleural effusion

c) What investigation should be performed to evaluate the pleural effusion? *(1 mark)*
   - Thoracocentesis

d) What tests are commonly performed on aspirated pleural fluid? *(7 marks)*
   - Cytology
   - Gram stain and culture
   - Fluid protein (including albumin)
   - Fluid lactate dehydrogenase (LDH)
   - Fluid pH
   - Fluid glucose
   - Fluid amylase

e) What is the purpose of Light's criteria? *(1 mark)*
   - To differentiate exudate from transudate

f) Which biochemical findings make an exudate more likely according to Light's criteria? *(3 marks)*
   - Pleural fluid protein to serum protein ratio >0.5
   - Pleural fluid LDH to serum LDH ratio >0.6
   - Pleural fluid LDH >$\frac{2}{3}$ of upper limit of normal for serum LDH
     (Data from Light RW, Macgregor MI, Luchsinger PC, Ball WC (1972). 'Pleural effusions: the diagnostic separation of transudates and exudates'. *Annals of Internal Medicine*, 77 (4): 507–13. doi:10.7326/0003-4819-77-4-507. PMID 4642731.)

g) How can the pleural fluid albumin concentration be useful in deciding if an exudate is likely? *(1 mark)*
   - [Serum albumin] – [effusion albumin] <1.2 g/dL is suggestive of exudate

h) What are the two most likely causes of this effusion? *(2 marks)*
   - Malignancy
   - Empyema

i) What would be the next therapeutic intervention? *(1 mark)*
   - Chest drain insertion

Further reading

Chapman S, Robinson G, Stradling J, West S, Wrightson J. Pleural effusion. In: *Oxford Handbook of Respiratory Medicine*, 3rd Edition, pp. 49–60. Oxford: Oxford University Press; 2014.

FFICM syllabus references 1.1, 2.2, 2.4, 2.6, 2.8, 3.1, 5.7.
CoBaTrICE domains 2, 3, 4, 5.

OSCE 6 station 7—data

Questions

a) What invasive methods are commonly used to measure intracranial pressure (ICP) after traumatic head injury? *(3 marks)*

b) According to Brain Trauma Foundation guidelines, at what level should a raised ICP be treated? *(1 mark)*

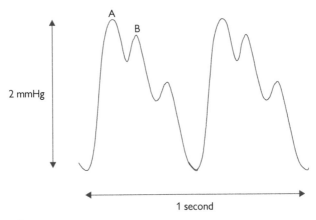

Figure 6.4 ICP waveform

Look at Figure 6.4.

c) In this normal ICP waveform, what are the main determinants of peaks A and B? *(2 marks)*

d) What would be a patient-related explanation for a waveform of reduced amplitude but unchanged morphology? *(1 mark)*

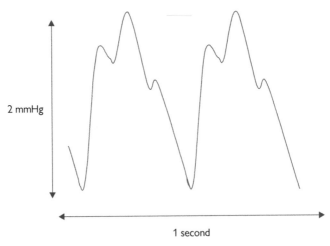

Figure 6.5 ICP waveform

Look at Figure 6.5.

e) What is the explanation for this change in waveform? *(2 marks)*

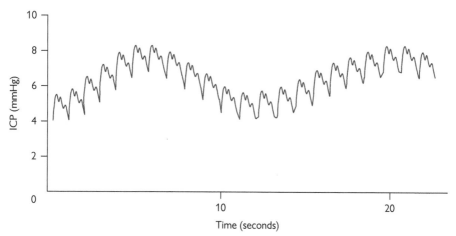

Figure 6.6 ICP waveform

Look at Figure 6.6.

f) What is the patient's heart rate? *(1 mark)*

g) What causes the sinusoidal slow waveform? *(1 mark)*

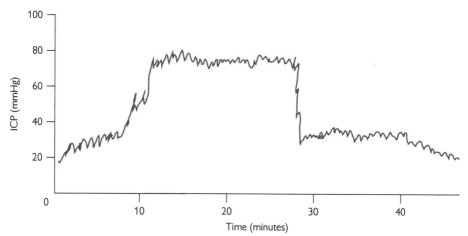

Figure 6.7 ICP waveform

Look at Figure 6.7.

h) What is shown here and what is the cause? *(3 marks)*

i) How do Lundberg A waves differ from Lundberg B waves? *(6 marks)*

Answers

a) What invasive methods are commonly used to measure intracranial pressure (ICP) after traumatic head injury? *(3 marks)*
- Intraventricular catheter
- Subdural pressure transducer
- Intraparenchymal monitor

(Lumbar cerebrospinal fluid (CSF) pressure monitoring is rarely used in the acute setting. Intracranial epidural catheters are another lesser used method.)

b) According to Brain Trauma Foundation guidelines, at what level should a raised ICP be treated? *(1 mark)*
- >22 mmHg

c) In this normal ICP waveform, what are the main determinants of peaks A and B? *(2 marks)*
- A—arterial pressure (transmitted via the choroid plexus)
- B—intracranial compliance

d) What would be a patient-related explanation for a waveform of reduced amplitude but unchanged morphology? *(1 mark)*
- Reduced CSF volume (e.g. after CSF drainage)

e) What is the explanation for this change in waveform? *(2 marks)*
- Reduced intracranial compliance ...
- ... because of intracranial hypertension

f) What is the patient's heart rate? *(1 mark)*
- Approximately 60 beats per minute

g) What causes the sinusoidal slow waveform? *(1 mark)*
- Respiration

h) What is shown here and what is the cause? *(3 marks)*
- Lundberg A wave (also known as a plateau wave)
- Caused by an increase in cerebral blood flow ...
- ... in response to a reduction in cerebral perfusion

i) How do Lundberg A waves differ from Lundberg B waves? *(6 marks)*

(1 mark for each heading and another for recall of specific details)
- Amplitude—A waves typically >50 mmHg, B waves typically 20–50 mmHg
- Duration—A waves approximately 5–20 minutes, B waves are shorter (approximately 1 minute)
- Pathophysiology—B waves are caused by unstable ICP (e.g. vasospasm), but can also be observed in non-pathological conditions (e.g. in rapid eye movement (REM) sleep). A waves are always pathological

Further reading

Brain Trauma Foundation. Guidelines for the management of severe traumatic brain injury, 4th edition. Available at https://braintrauma.org/uploads/03/12/Guidelines_for_Management_of_Severe_TBI_4th_Edition.pdf [accessed 14 January 2020].

Czosnyka M, Pickard JD. Monitoring and interpretation of intracranial pressure. *Journal of Neurology, Neurosurgery, and Psychiatry* 2004;75:813–821.

Smith M. Monitoring intracranial pressure in traumatic brain injury. *Anesthesia & Analgesia* 2008;106:240–248.

FFICM syllabus references 1.5, 2.2, 2.7, 3.6.
CoBaTrICE domain 2.

OSCE 6 station 8—data

Questions

A 27-year-old man has fallen from a ladder. He has obvious bilateral femoral deformities and diffuse pelvic tenderness. There is no external bleeding. The findings of the primary survey include the following:

- Maintained and patent airway
- Normal chest auscultation with saturations of 97% on high-flow oxygen
- Systolic blood pressure of 76 mmHg, heart rate of 110 beats per minute (regular)
- Glasgow Coma Scale score 15

a) What sources of haemorrhage should be considered? *(4 marks)*
b) Why should a pelvic spring test not be performed? *(1 mark)*
c) What investigation, performed in the resuscitation area, may help in planning how to control the bleeding? *(1 mark)*

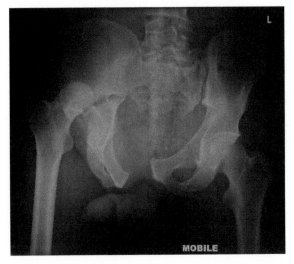

Figure 6.8 Pelvis X-ray
Reproduced from *Oxford Textbook of Fundamentals of Surgery*, Thomas WEG et al., Figure 6.4.1. © 2016 Oxford University Press. Reproduced with permission of the Licensor through PLSclear

A focused assessment with sonography in trauma (FAST) scan shows no sign of intraperitoneal bleeding. A pelvic X-ray is performed (Figure 6.8).

d) What does the X-ray show? *(3 marks)*
e) What procedures should be performed to improve haemodynamic stability? *(2 marks)*
f) Aside from blood products, what other haemostatic therapy should be given? *(1 mark)*
g) What are the potential mechanisms of bleeding in an open book pelvic injury? *(2 marks)*

The patient remains haemodynamically unstable despite a massive transfusion of blood and blood products, application of a pelvic binder, and femoral traction. A computed tomography (CT) scan is performed.

h) What additional information might the CT scan give regarding the pelvic injury and the haemodynamic instability? *(2 marks)*

The CT scan does not identify any non-pelvic sources of bleeding, but a contrast 'blush' is seen.

i) What intervention should be performed to achieve haemodynamic stability? *(1 mark)*

The patient is haemodynamically stable after angiographic embolization and surgery is planned to fix his pelvic and femoral fractures.

j) What other injuries related to the pelvic fracture should be considered? *(3 marks)*

Answers

a) What sources of haemorrhage should be considered? *(4 marks)*
-   Unstable pelvic fracture
-   Intra-abdominal bleeding
-   Bilateral femoral fractures
-   Haemothorax

b) Why should a pelvic spring test not be performed? *(1 mark)*
-   This may disrupt the 'first clot' and precipitate further bleeding

c) What investigation, performed in the resuscitation area, may help in planning how to control the bleeding? *(1 mark)*
-   A FAST (focused assessment with sonography in trauma) scan

d) What does the X-ray show? *(3 marks)*
-   Right acetabular fracture
-   Open book pelvic fracture
-   Dislocated right hip

e) What procedures should be performed to improve haemodynamic stability? *(2 marks)*
-   Application of a pelvic binder
-   Femoral traction

f) Aside from blood products, what other haemostatic therapy should be given? *(1 mark)*
-   Tranexamic acid

g) What are the potential mechanisms of bleeding in an open book pelvic injury? *(2 marks)*

(1 mark per mechanism to a maximum of 2)
-   Tearing of posterior venous plexuses
-   Pelvic arterial bleeding
-   Cancellous bone fragment bleeding

h) What additional information might the CT scan give regarding the pelvic injury and the haemodynamic instability? *(2 marks)*

(1 mark per correct answer to a maximum of 2)
-   To quantify the extent and location of any retroperitoneal bleeding
-   Contrast 'blush' may help locate an active bleeding site
-   To identify other sources of bleeding which may have been missed on the FAST scan
-   To aid surgical planning for pelvic fixation

i) What intervention should be performed to achieve haemodynamic stability? *(1 mark)*
-   Angiographic embolization of the bleeding vessel

j) What other injuries related to the pelvic fracture should be considered? *(3 marks)*
-   Neurological injury
-   Bowel injury
-   Bladder or urethral injury

Notes

Although this question gives the appearance of being about pelvic fractures, it is really about general principles of bleeding in trauma. Even if a topic is unfamiliar on first encounter, you should apply your general knowledge and principles for maximum marks.

Further reading

Rossaint R, Bouillon B, Cerny V, Coats TJ, Duranteau J, Fernández-Mondéjar E, et al. The European guideline on management of major bleeding and coagulopathy following trauma: fourth edition. *Critical Care* 2016;20:100.

FFICM syllabus references 1.5, 2.1, 2.2, 2.6, 3.3.
CoBaTrICE domains 1, 2, 4, 5.

OSCE 6 station 9—data

Questions

A 71-year-old man presented with a fever of 38.7°C and symptoms of malaise and fatigue. A new murmur had been heard, so a transthoracic echocardiogram was arranged.

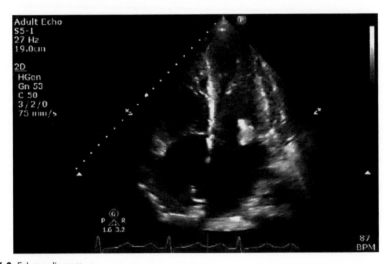

Figure 6.9 Echocardiogram
© Oxford University Hospitals NHS Foundation Trust 2016, with permission

Look at Figure 6.9.

a) What abnormality is present on this apical four-chamber view? *(2 marks)*
b) What is the diagnosis? *(1 mark)*
c) Which groups of bacteria most commonly cause infective endocarditis (IE) on native valves? *(3 marks)*
d) What is the name of the criteria used to diagnose IE? *(1 mark)*
e) What are the clinical criteria for diagnosis of definite IE using the modified Duke classification? *(8 marks)*
f) Which microorganisms are predictors of poor outcomes in infective endocarditis? *(2 marks)*
g) What are the groups of indications for surgery in native left-sided valve endocarditis? *(3 marks)*

Answers

a) What abnormality is present on this apical four-chamber view? *(2 marks)*
   - An echogenic mass …
   - … on the mitral valve
b) What is the diagnosis? *(1 mark)*
   - Infective endocarditis
c) Which groups of bacteria most commonly cause infective endocarditis (IE) on native valves? *(3 marks)*
   - Staphylococci
   - Streptococci
   - Enterococci
d) What is the name of the criteria used to diagnose IE? *(1 mark)*
   - Modified Duke criteria
e) What are the clinical criteria for diagnosis of definite IE using the modified Duke classification? *(8 marks)*

   - Major criteria:
     - Positive blood cultures:
       - Microorganisms consistent with IE from two separate blood cultures
       - Microorganisms consistent with IE from persistently positive blood cultures
     - Evidence of endocardial involvement, demonstrated by a positive echocardiogram
   - Minor criteria:
     - Predisposing factor: known cardiac lesion, recreational drug injection
     - Fever >38°C
     - Evidence of embolism: arterial emboli, pulmonary infarcts, Janeway lesions, conjunctival haemorrhage
     - Immunological problems: glomerulonephritis, Osler's nodes, Roth's spots, positive rheumatoid factor
     - Microbiological evidence: positive blood culture (that doesn't meet a major criterion) or serological evidence of infection with organism consistent with IE but not satisfying major criteria
   - Two major criteria, one major and three minor criteria, or five minor criteria confirm the diagnosis
   (Data from Li JS, Sexton DJ et al. Proposed modifications to the Duke criteria for the diagnosis of infective endocarditis. *Clinical Infectious Diseases.* 2000 Apr; 30(4): 633–638.)
f) Which microorganisms are predictors of poor outcome in patients with infective endocarditis? *(2 marks)*

   (1 mark for each organism to a maximum of 2)
   - *Staphylococcus aureus*
   - Fungi
   - Non-HACEK Gram-negative bacilli
g) What are the indications for surgery in native left-sided valve endocarditis? *(3 marks)*
   - Heart failure
   - Uncontrolled infection—persistent/progressing/perivalvular extension
   - Prevention of embolism

Further reading

Habib G, Lancellotti P, Antunes MJ, Bongiorni MG, Casalta JP, Del Zotti F, et al. 2015 ESC Guidelines for the management of infective endocarditis: the Task Force for the Management of Infective Endocarditis of the European Society of Cardiology (ESC). *European Heart Journal* 2015;36:3075–3128.

FFICM syllabus references 2.2, 2.4, 2.6, 2.8, 3.1, 3.9.
CoBaTrICE domains 2, 3.

OSCE 6 station 10—data

Questions

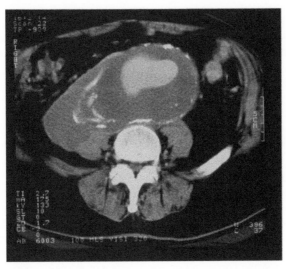

Figure 6.10 CT abdomen

Reproduced from *Oxford Textbook of Vascular Surgery*, Thompson MM *et al.*, Figure 7.4.19. © 2016 Oxford University Press. Reproduced with permission of the Licensor through PLSclear

A 75-year-old man has presented to the emergency department with back pain and shock. A computed tomography (CT) scan is performed (Figure 6.10).

a) What is the diagnosis? *(1 mark)*

b) What surgical options are available for the treatment of a ruptured abdominal aortic aneurysm? *(2 marks)*

c) What are the risk factors for development of an atherosclerotic abdominal aortic aneurysm? *(6 marks)*

d) When predicting outcome post repair of a ruptured aortic aneurysm, what variables are used to calculate the Glasgow Aneurysm Score? *(5 marks)*

An open surgical repair of the aneurysm is performed. Six hours postoperatively the patient's lactate has risen from 6 to 12 mmol/L despite optimal fluid therapy and vasoactive drug support.

e) What complications should be considered? *(3 marks)*

f) What are the potential mechanisms of ischaemic colitis post abdominal aortic aneurysm repair? *(3 marks)*

Answers

a) What is the diagnosis? *(1 mark)*
 • Ruptured abdominal aortic aneurysm
b) What surgical options are available for the treatment of a ruptured aortic aneurysm? *(2 marks)*
 • Open repair
 • Endovascular repair (EVAR)
c) What are the risk factors for development of an atherosclerotic abdominal aortic aneurysm? *(6 marks)*
 • Male sex
 • Increased age
 • Hypertension
 • Smoking
 • Hypercholesterolaemia
 • Family history
d) When predicting outcome post repair of a ruptured aortic aneurysm, what variables are used to calculate the Glasgow Aneurysm Score? *(5 marks)*
 • Presence of shock
 • Age
 • Pre-existing myocardial disease
 • Pre-existing cerebrovascular disease
 • Pre-existing renal disease
e) What complications should be considered? *(3 marks)*
 • Mesenteric ischaemia
 • Limb or buttock ischaemia
 • Perioperative cardiac event
f) What are the potential mechanisms of ischaemic colitis post abdominal aortic aneurysm repair? *(3 marks)*
 • Systemic hypoperfusion
 • Embolic ischaemia
 • Surgical ligation

Further reading

Swerdlow NJ, Wu WW, Schermerhorn ML. Open and endovascular management of aortic aneurysms. *Circulation Research* 2019;124:647–661.

FFICM syllabus references 2.2, 2.6, 3.3, 6.1.
CoBaTrICE domains 1, 2, 6.

OSCE 6 station 11—data

Questions

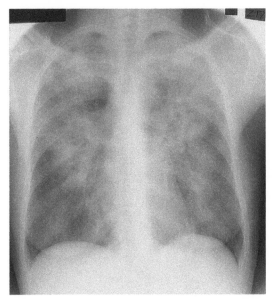

Figure 6.11 Chest X-ray

Reproduced from *Oxford Textbook of Medicine, Fifth Edition*, Warrell D, et al., Figure 18.14.1.1. © 2010 Oxford University Press. Reproduced with permission of the Licensor through PLSclear

A 65-year-old smoker with moderate chronic obstructive pulmonary disease has been admitted with breathlessness and haemoptysis (1200 mL in the last 10 hours). She is tachypnoeic (respiratory rate 30 breaths per minute) and her SpO_2 is 92% with supplemental oxygen. Her heart rate is 110 beats per minute (sinus rhythm) and her blood pressure is 88/65 mmHg.

Look at Figure 6.11.

a) What is the most striking abnormality on the chest X-ray? *(1 mark)*

b) What are the most common causes of death in massive pulmonary haemorrhage (MPH)? *(2 marks)*

c) From which vessels does bleeding most commonly arise in MPH? *(1 mark)*

d) What are the treatment priorities in MPH? *(5 marks)*

e) What investigations are used to identify the source of bleeding in MPH? *(4 marks)*

The patient is admitted to critical care and invasively ventilated due to worsening respiratory failure.

f) What bronchoscopic interventions are available at the bedside to stop bleeding in MPH? *(3 marks)*

g) What therapeutic options are used to stop bleeding in MPH where there is no visible source at bronchoscopy? *(2 marks)*

h) What are the serious complications of bronchial artery embolization? *(2 marks)*

Answers

a) What is the most striking abnormality on the chest X-ray? *(1 mark)*
  - Bilateral air space shadowing predominately in the mid and upper zones
b) What are the most common causes of death in massive pulmonary haemorrhage (MPH)? *(2 marks)*
  - Asphyxia
  - Haemorrhagic shock
c) From which vessels does bleeding most commonly arise in MPH? *(1 mark)*
  - Bronchial arteries
d) What are the treatment priorities in MPH? *(5 marks)*
  - Administration of oxygen and airway protection
  - Resuscitation with blood products to restore circulating blood volume and correct coagulopathy
  - Lung isolation in unilateral disease to ensure adequate gas exchange and avoid contamination of the unaffected lung
  - Identify the source of bleeding
  - Stop the bleeding
e) What investigations are used to identify the source of bleeding in MPH? *(4 marks)*
  - Chest X-ray
  - Flexible or rigid bronchoscopy
  - Computed tomography
  - Angiography
f) What bronchoscopic interventions are available at the bedside to stop bleeding in MPH? *(3 marks)*
  - Pulmonary lavage with cold saline
  - Topical medications—vasoconstrictors (e.g. adrenaline), antidiuretic hormone derivatives, procoagulants (e.g. fibrinogen-thrombin)
  - Balloon tamponade with an endobronchial blocker or a Fogarty balloon catheter
g) What therapeutic options are used to stop bleeding in MPH where there is no visible source at bronchoscopy? *(2 marks)*
  - Endovascular embolization
  - Surgical excision of lung segments
h) What are the most serious complications of bronchial artery embolization? *(2 marks)*
  - Bronchial artery wall necrosis and rupture
  - Spinal cord ischaemia

Further reading

Larici AR, Franchi P, Occhipinti M, Contegiacomo A, del Ciello A, Calandriello L, et al. Diagnosis and management of haemoptysis. *Diagnostic and Interventional Radiology* 2014;20:299–309.
Sakr L, Dutau H. Massive haemorrhage: an update on the role of bronchoscopy in diagnosis and management. *Respiration* 2010;80:38–58.

FFICM syllabus references 2.2, 2.6, 3.1, 3.8.
CoBaTrICE domains 1, 2, 3, 4.

OSCE 6 station 12—equipment

Questions

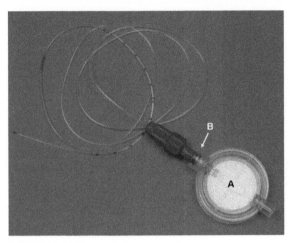

Figure 6.12 Medical device

Reproduced from *Principles and Practice of Regional Anaesthesia, Fourth Edition*, McLeod G, McCartney C, and Wildsmith T, Figure 14.3. © 2012 Oxford University Press. Reproduced with permission of the Licensor through PLSclear

Look at Figure 6.12.

a) What is A? *(1 mark)*

b) What would you do if an epidural catheter became disconnected at point B? *(1 mark)*

c) What safety measures are employed to minimize incorrect drug administration via an epidural? *(6 marks)*

You are asked to review a patient on the high dependency unit who is complaining of pain following open upper abdominal surgery. A thoracic epidural was inserted by the anaesthetist at the level of T10 achieving good analgesia until 3 hours previously.

An infusion of 0.125% levo-bupivacaine and 2 mcg/mL of fentanyl is running at 5 mL/hour with a patient-controlled epidural analgesia (PCEA) bolus of 5 mL available up to every 20 minutes.

Nursing assessment reveals a thermal sensory block level at the umbilicus on the right and the xiphisternum on the left.

d) At what dermatomal level is the xiphisternum? *(1 mark)*

e) At what dermatomal level is the umbilicus? *(1 mark)*

f) What factors affect the cephalad distribution of neural blockade during thoracic epidural analgesia? *(4 marks)*

The patient receives an epidural bolus of 10 mL of the maintenance epidural infusate and the background rate is increased to 8 mL/hour. You are asked to reassess the patient an hour later as routine monitoring reveals a dense bilateral motor block.

g) What are the differential diagnoses of a dense motor block in a patient with an epidural? *(4 marks)*

h) What would your initial management be in this case? *(1 mark)*

The motor block has not regressed after 3 hours despite turning the epidural infusion off.

i) What investigation should be performed to exclude an epidural haematoma? *(1 mark)*

Answers

a) What is A? *(1 mark)*
   - A bacterial and microscopic particle filter

b) What would you do if an epidural catheter became disconnected at point B? *(1 mark)*
   - Remove the catheter

c) What safety measures are employed to minimize incorrect drug administration via an epidural? *(6 marks)*

   (1 mark per feature to a maximum of 6)
   - Medication:
     - Use of pre-prepared infusions labelled for epidural use only
     - Storing epidural infusions separately from parenteral medications
   - Equipment:
     - Use of dedicated epidural equipment with programmed protocols that undergo regular maintenance
     - Locking infusion devices to prevent programme adjustments/tampering
     - Use of dedicated and easily identifiable epidural administration sets
     - Use of a closed epidural infusion with no injection ports in the circuit between the pump and the patient, preventing bolus drug administration
     - Use of non-Luer lock connectors
   - Staff:
     - Mandatory training and competency-based assessment

d) At what dermatomal level is the xiphisternum? *(1 mark)*
   - T6

e) At what dermatomal level is the umbilicus? *(1 mark)*
   - T10

f) What factors affect the cephalad distribution of neural blockade during thoracic epidural analgesia? *(4 marks)*

   (1 mark per factor to a maximum of 4)
   - Non-patient factors:
     - Level of catheter insertion
     - Epidural catheter tip position
     - Mass and volume of drug injected
   - Patient factors:
     - Age
     - Increased intra-abdominal pressure
     - Epidural adhesions
     - Patient position

g) What are the differential diagnoses of a dense motor block in a patient with an epidural? *(4 marks)*
   - Effect of a large bolus of local anaesthetic
   - Migration of the catheter into the subarachnoid or extradural space
   - Epidural abscess
   - Epidural haematoma

h) What would your management be of a patient with a dense motor block? *(1 mark)*
   - Stop the epidural infusion

i) What investigation should be performed to exclude an epidural haematoma? *(1 mark)*
   - Emergency magnetic resonance imaging of the spine

Notes

This question will be more straightforward for those with an anaesthetics background, but the management of epidural analgesia is required knowledge for everybody.

Further reading

Cook TM, Counsell D, Wilsmith JAW, Royal College of Anaesthesia. Major complications of central neuraxial block: report on the Third National Audit Project of the Royal College of Anaesthetists. *British Journal of Anaesthesia* 2009;102:179–190.

Faculty of Pain Medicine of the Royal College of Anaesthetists. Best practice in the management of epidural analgesia in the hospital setting. 2010. Available at: https://www.britishpainsociety.org/static/uploads/resources/files/pub_prof_EpiduralAnalgesia2010.pdf [accessed 14 January 2020].

Visser WA, Lee RA, Gielen MJM. Factors affecting the distribution of neural blockade by local anaesthetics in epidural anaesthesia and a comparison of lumbar versus thoracic epidural anaesthesia. *Anaesthesia and Analgesia* 2008;107:708–721.

FFICM syllabus references 4.1, 5.16, 7.2.
CoBaTrICE domains 6, 7.

OSCE 6 station 13—equipment

Questions

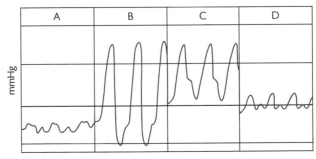

Figure 6.13 Waveform
Reproduced from *Emergencies in Anaesthesia, Second Edition*, Allman KG et al., Figure 14.27. © 2009 Oxford University Press. Reproduced with permission of the Licensor through PLSclear

Look at Figure 6.13.

a) This is a waveform from an invasive monitoring device, what is the device? *(1 mark)*

During pulmonary artery catheter (PAC) insertion, a series of distinct waveforms are seen.

b) What anatomical positions do waveforms A–D represent? *(4 marks)*

c) When advancing the PAC through an inducer sheath in the right internal jugular vein, at what skin depth would you expect to see the right ventricular, pulmonary artery, and pulmonary artery occlusion pressure (PAOP) waveforms in an average-sized adult male? *(3 marks)*

d) What characteristics of waveform C support the successful movement of the catheter tip into the pulmonary artery? *(3 marks)*

e) If during PAC insertion you have advanced the PAC over 50 cm (in an average-sized adult with a right internal jugular insertion) and the waveform has not changed from waveform B to C, what would you do and why? *(4 marks)*

f) What is the optimal position of the PAC tip on a chest X-ray? *(1 mark)*

g) What error in PAOP measurement may occur if the PAC tip is in an apical position on chest X-ray? *(1 mark)*

h) What are the complications specifically related to PAC insertion and advancement (excluding central venous access)? *(3 marks)*

Answers

a) This is a waveform from an invasive monitoring device, what is the device? (*1 mark*)
   - Pulmonary artery catheter
b) What anatomical positions do waveforms A–D represent? (*4 marks*)
   - Waveform A = right atrial pressure
   - Waveform B = right ventricular (RV) pressure
   - Waveform C = pulmonary artery (PA) pressure
   - Waveform D = PA occlusion pressure (PAOP—also known as PA wedge pressure or PA capillary pressure)
c) When advancing the PAC through an inducer sheath in the right internal jugular vein, at what skin depth would you expect to see the right ventricular, pulmonary artery, and pulmonary artery occlusion pressure (PAOP) waveforms in an average-sized adult male? (*3 marks*)
   - RV—25–30 cm
   - PA—5–10 cm beyond RV, i.e. 35–40 cm
   - PAOP—10 cm beyond PA, i.e. approximately 45 cm
d) What characteristics of waveform C support the successful movement of the catheter tip into the pulmonary artery? (*3 marks*)
   - Presence of the dicrotic notch
   - Rise in diastolic pressure from baseline
   - Down-sloping diastolic wave
e) If during PAC insertion you have advanced the PAC over 50 cm (in an average sized adult with a right internal jugular insertion) and the waveform has not changed from waveform B to C, what would you do and why? (*4 marks*)
   - Deflate the balloon ...
   - ... and withdraw the catheter ...
   - ... to avoid coiling or knotting of the catheter in the RV ...
   - ... and injury to intracardiac structures
f) What is the optimal position of the PAC tip on a chest X-ray? (*1 mark*)
   - The PAC tip should be below the level of the left atrium
g) What error in PAOP measurement may occur if the PAC tip is in an apical position on chest X-ray? (*1 mark*)
   - PAOP will be overestimated, reflecting the alveolar pressure which exceeds capillary pressure
h) What complications are associated with PAC use and maintenance? (*3 marks*)

   (1 mark per complication to a maximum of 3)
   - PA damage, e.g. pseudoaneurysm or perforation
   - Pulmonary infarction due to migration of the catheter tip into a distal branch of the PA
   - Thrombosis
   - Infection—catheter-related bloodstream infection and endocarditis
   - Venous air embolism

Further reading

PAC-MAN study group. Pulmonary artery catheters in patient management. *Lancet* 2005;366;472–477.

FFICM syllabus references 2.2, 2.7, 5.14.
CoBaTrICE domain 2.

OSCE 7

OSCE 7 station 1—professionalism

Questions

Mrs Smith was admitted to the intensive care unit 5 days ago with community-acquired pneumonia and an obstructing lung tumour. Her condition has continued to worsen over this time, such that she is now clearly dying despite full active treatment (which consists of maximal invasive ventilation and large doses of vasopressors and inotropic medication). The healthcare team all agree that there is no chance of survival and that there are no other treatment options available.

You have been asked to speak to her family to explain that life-sustaining treatment will be withdrawn.

a) What will you say to the family? *(10 marks)*

The family accept that death is inevitable and ask what will happen next.

b) What will you say? *(5 marks)*

Answers

a) What will you say to the family? *(10 marks)*
  - Introduce yourself
  - Establish the relationships of those in the room and how they want to be addressed
  - Ask if they would like anyone else to be present
  - Ask what is already known and recap events to date
  - Use a warning shot
  - Explain deterioration despite full efforts and the collective professional opinion that death is inevitable
  - Explain you are not asking the family to decide whether life-sustaining treatment should be withdrawn
  - Use the term 'will die'
  - Check understanding of what has been said
  - Offer the opportunity for further discussion

b) What will you say? *(5 marks)*
  - Specify what treatment will be withdrawn (e.g. stopping infusions, extubation)
  - Ask about any expressed end of life wishes
  - Mention symptom control and comfort at the end of life
  - Offer additional support, e.g. religious
  - Close the discussion

General communication *(5 marks)*
  Marks awarded for behaviours such as the following:

  - Display active listening—nodding, verbal affirmations, etc.
  - Display empathy—verbalize the awfulness of the situation
  - Use silences and pauses effectively, appropriate pace of speech
  - Avoid medical jargon
  - Avoid euphemisms

Notes

The purpose of this question is to give a framework for end of life discussions. For clarity, a whole script has not been included but the mark scheme should give an idea of what should be covered. The separation into two questions is somewhat arbitrary, but it ensures a conversation about end of life care is prompted.

Further reading

Rocker G, Puntillo KA, Azoulay E, Nelson JE, Watson M. Withholding and withdrawal of life support. In: Rocker G, Puntillo K, Azoulay E, Nelson J (eds.) *End of Life Care in the ICU: From Advanced Disease to Bereavement*, pp. 241–280. Oxford: Oxford University Press; 2010.

FFICM syllabus references 7.1, 12.1, 12.4.
CoBaTrICE domains 8, 12.

OSCE 7 station 2—resuscitation

Questions

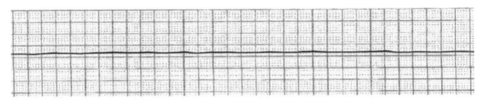

Figure 7.1 Rhythm strip
Reproduced from *Care of the Acutely Ill Adult: An Essential Guide for Nurses*, Creed F and Spiers C, Figure 13.16 © 2010 Oxford University Press. Reproduced with permission of the Licensor through PLSclear

A patient has had a cardiac arrest on the delivery suite after complaining of severe breathlessness and chest pain. She was labouring normally without medical intervention, and examination 2 hours earlier found her cervix to be 7 cm dilated. The only medications she had received was Entonox® for analgesia.

She has no previous medical history and had uneventful antenatal care.

On your arrival, basic life support is being delivered and the defibrillator pads are being applied. A rhythm strip has been printed (Figure 7.1).

a) What is the rhythm? *(1 mark)*
b) Outline how you would proceed *(14 marks)*
c) During resuscitation, the midwife asks 'Are there any differences in performing chest compressions in the pregnant patient?' *(1 mark)*

At the end of 2 minutes of cardiopulmonary resuscitation (CPR) the rhythm is unchanged.

d) During the second cycle of CPR the anaesthetic consultant arrives and asks 'What is going on?' *(4 marks)*

Answers

a) What is the rhythm? *(1 mark)*
  - Asystole
b) Outline how you would proceed *(14 marks)*
  - Confirm cardiorespiratory arrest and continue CPR
  - Call for senior obstetric, anaesthetic, and neonatal support via the maternal cardiac arrest call
  - Manually displace the uterus or perform left tilt to 15–30 degrees by insertion of a wedge
  - Continue high-quality CPR with minimal interruptions (<5 seconds) at a ratio of 30 cardiac compressions to 2 ventilation breaths with supplementary oxygen
  - Establish intravenous (IV) access and administer 1 mg of adrenaline IV followed by a saline flush
  - Evaluate the reversible causes of cardiac arrest:
    - Hypoxia—plan for endotracheal intubation
    - Hypothermia—check temperature
    - Hypovolaemia—check for vaginal bleeding and give a fluid bolus
    - Hypo/hyperkalaemia or glycaemia—check recent bloods and capillary glucose
    - Toxins—check drug prescription chart
    - Tension pneumothorax—auscultate chest during ventilation
    - Cardiac tamponade—look for distended neck veins
    - Thromboembolic disease—look for signs of deep vein thrombosis
  - Consider perimortem caesarean
c) During resuscitation, the midwife asks 'Are there any differences in performing chest compressions in the pregnant patient?' *(1 mark)*
  - Hand position for chest compressions may need to be higher on the sternum in the third trimester
d) During the second cycle of CPR, the anaesthetic consultant arrives and asks 'What is going on?' *(4 marks)*
  - Situation—this is the second cycle of CPR in an asystolic cardiac arrest
  - Background—the patient is a healthy 39-week pregnant women who was labouring uneventfully until she complained of chest pain and breathlessness immediately prior to cardiac arrest
  - Assessment—there has been no response to initial resuscitation attempts and no reversible cause identified
  - Recommendation—caesarean section should be undertaken while resuscitation of the mother continues

Notes

During the resuscitation station there may be a task that you want to perform that would take up too much time or test a skill that is not the focus of the station. In this scenario it is intubation, but other examples could be performing a bedside echocardiogram, inserting a chest drain, etc.

The way the examiners usually get around this is to say that equipment is not immediately available, or that someone else will perform the task in due course. You will still score the marks for stating what you want to do, but don't get preoccupied by the fact you can't do it.

Further reading

Truhlar A, Deakin CD, Soar J, Khalifa GEA, Alfonzo A, Bierens JJLM, et al. European Resuscitation Council Guidelines for Resuscitation 2015: Section 4: cardiac arrest in special circumstances. *Resuscitation* 2015; 95:148–201.

FFICM syllabus references 1.2, 2.3, 3.11.
CoBaTrICE domains 1, 2, 3, 4.

OSCE 7 station 3—data

Questions

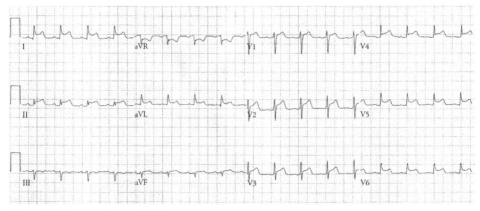

Figure 7.2 Electrocardiogram (ECG)

Reproduced from *The Brigham Intensive Review of Internal Medicine*, Singh AK and Loscalzo J, Figure 81.1. © 2014 Oxford University Press. Reproduced with permission of the Licensor through PLSclear

A 60-year-old man underwent a third catheter ablation procedure for persistent atrial fibrillation (AF). He was discharged in sinus rhythm. Ten days later he was admitted to the emergency department with chest pain that is worse on inspiration. His electrocardiogram (ECG) is shown in Figure 7.2.

a) Around which structure is ablation performed during a first procedure for AF? *(1 mark)*

b) What finding on transthoracic echocardiography would be a contraindication to catheter ablation? *(1 mark)*

c) What is the most striking abnormality on this ECG and what is the diagnosis? *(2 marks)*

d) Which four clinical features are used to diagnose pericarditis? *(4 marks)*

e) Apart from ST elevation, what other ECG abnormalities can be present during the early stage of pericarditis? *(2 marks)*

f) Why is performing an echocardiogram useful in pericarditis? *(2 marks)*

g) What medications are commonly used for symptomatic relief in pericarditis? *(3 marks)*

One week later, the patient re-presents with fever, worsening chest pain, malaise, and dysphagia. Following an episode of haematemesis, a diagnosis of atrio-oesophageal fistula (AOF) is suspected.

h) Which imaging investigation should be performed if an AOF is suspected? *(1 mark)*

i) What would be the risks of upper gastrointestinal endoscopy in this patient? *(2 marks)*

j) What is the treatment of choice for an AOF? *(1 mark)*

k) How can catheter ablation for AF cause an AOF? *(1 mark)*

Answers

a) Around which structure is ablation performed during a first procedure for AF? *(1 mark)*
   - Pulmonary vein
b) What finding on transthoracic echocardiography would be a contraindication to catheter ablation? *(1 mark)*
   - Left atrial thrombus
c) What is the abnormality on this ECG and what is the diagnosis? *(2 marks)*
   - Diffuse concave ST-segment elevation
   - Pericarditis
d) Which four clinical features are used to diagnose pericarditis? *(4 marks)*
   - Characteristic chest pain—typically sharp and pleuritic improved by sitting up and leaning forward
   - Pericardial friction rub on auscultation
   - Typical ECG changes
   - New or worsening pericardial effusion
e) Apart from ST elevation, what other ECG abnormalities can be present during the early stage of pericarditis? *(2 marks)*
   - ST depression in AVR and V1
   - R-wave depression
f) Why is performing an echocardiogram useful in pericarditis? *(2 marks)*
   - To identify if a pericardial effusion is present
   - To assess for the presence of concurrent myocarditis
g) What medications are commonly used for symptomatic relief in pericarditis? *(3 marks)*
   - Non-steroidal anti-inflammatory drugs
   - Corticosteroids
   - Colchicine
h) Which imaging investigation should be performed if an AOF is suspected? *(1 mark)*
   - Contrast computed tomography of the chest
i) What would be the risks of upper gastrointestinal endoscopy in this patient? *(2 marks)*
   - Torrential bleeding
   - Air embolism
j) What is the treatment of choice for an AOF? *(1 mark)*
   - Urgent surgical repair
k) How can catheter ablation for AF cause an AOF? *(1 mark)*
   - The thin-walled left atrium lies immediately anterior to the oesophagus and any energy or heat transmitted during the procedure can cause ulceration and necrosis, which can in turn erode into the left atrium

Notes

In an exam, being asked about a rare condition you haven't heard of (such as AOF) might throw you. This question demonstrates that the marks allocated to the weird and wonderful won't be the majority. Also, the questions asked about a rare topic will be straightforward (e.g. stem j), testing other knowledge (e.g. stem k, which is really an anatomy question), or can be worked out from first principles and common sense (e.g. stem i).

Further reading

Han HC, Ha FJ, Sanders P, Spencer R, Teh AW, O'Donnell D, et al. Atrioesophageal fistula: clinical presentation, procedural characteristics, diagnostic investigations, and treatment outcomes. *Circulation: Arrhythmia and Electrophysiology* 2017;10:e005579.

FFICM syllabus references 2.1, 2.2, 2.3, 3.1.
CoBaTrICE domains 2, 3.

OSCE 7 station 4—data

Questions

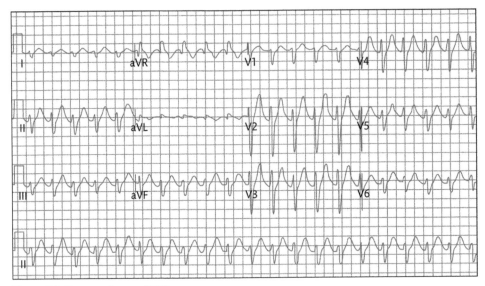

Figure 7.3 Electrocardiogram (ECG)

Reproduced from *Challenging Concepts in Emergency Medicine: Cases with Expert Commentary*, Thenabadu S et al., Figure 14.1. © 2015 Oxford University Press. Reproduced with permission of the Licensor through PLSclear

You are asked to review a 20-year-old woman in the emergency department. She has presented having taken a large overdose of her mother's regular medication. Her mother is treated for hypertension and depression. Her electrocardiogram (ECG) is shown in Figure 7.3.

a) What abnormalities are present on the ECG? *(5 marks)*

An arterial blood gas (ABG) test shows the following (normal ranges in brackets):

- pH 7.30 (7.35–7.45)
- PCO_2 4.9 kPa (4.7–6.0 kPa)
- PO_2 29.5 kPa (>10.6 kPa)
- HCO_3^- 17 mmol/L (24–30 mmol/L)
- Base excess −9 mmol/L (±2 mmol/L)

b) What abnormality is shown by the ABG results? *(1 mark)*

c) Which class of drugs would be most likely to explain the ECG and ABG findings in this case? *(1 mark)*

d) By what mechanisms do tricyclic antidepressants (TCAs) exhibit their toxic effects? *(4 marks)*

e) What is the most commonly used treatment for TCA overdose? *(1 mark)*

f) In the absence of acidosis, under what circumstances should the use of hypertonic 8.4% sodium bicarbonate be considered? *(3 marks)*

g) Complete the blanks in Table 7.1q *(5 marks)*

Table 7.1q Toxins and their antidotes

Toxin	Antidote
	Oxygen
Lidocaine	
	Glucagon, atropine
Cyanide	
	Glucose, octreotide

Answers

a) What abnormalities are present in the ECG? (*5 marks*)
- Sinus tachycardia, 130 beats per minute
- Extreme axis deviation
- Widened QRS
- Prominent R wave in aVR
- Absent P waves

b) What abnormality is shown by the ABG results? (*1 mark*)
- Metabolic acidosis

c) Which class of drugs would be most likely to explain the ECG and ABG findings in this case? (*1 mark*)
- Tricyclic antidepressants

d) By what mechanisms do tricyclic antidepressants (TCAs) exhibit their toxic effects? (*4 marks*)
- Anticholinergic action
- Inhibition of noradrenaline and serotonergic reuptake at nerve terminals
- Direct alpah -adrenergic blockade
- Membrane stabilizing effect on the myocardium by blockade of the cardiac and neurological fast sodium channels

e) What is the most commonly used treatment for TCA overdose? (*1 mark*)
- Hypertonic 8.4% sodium bicarbonate

f) In the absence of acidosis, under what circumstances should the use of hypertonic 8.4% sodium bicarbonate be considered? (*3 marks*)
- QRS duration >100 ms
- Arrhythmias
- Hypotension resistant to fluid resuscitation

g) Complete the blanks in Table 7.1a (*5 marks*)

Table 7.1a Toxins and their antidotes

Toxin	Antidote
Carbon monoxide	Oxygen
Lidocaine	Intralipid
Beta blockers	Glucagon, atropine
Cyanide	Dicobalt edetate or sodium nitrite with sodium thiosulphate
Sulphonylureas	Glucose, octreotide

Further reading

Body R, Bartram T, Azam F, Mackway-Jones K. Guidelines in Emergency Medicine Network (GEMNet): guideline for the management of tricyclic antidepressant overdose. *Emergency Medicine Journal* 2011;28:347–368.

Rao S, Townsend E. Tricyclic antidepressant overdose. In: Thenabadu S, Cantle F, Lacy C (eds.) *Challenging Concepts in Emergency Medicine: Cases with Expert Commentary*, pp. 137–146. Oxford: Oxford University Press; 2015.

FFICM syllabus references 1.1, 2.2, 2.3, 2.5, 2.8, 3.1, 3.3, 3.10, 4.1, 4.8.
CoBaTrICE domains 1, 2, 3.

OSCE 7 station 5—data

Questions

a) What are the potential benefits of conducting research in the NHS? *(3 marks)*
b) Match each of the research roles to their correct description *(4 marks)*
   1. Principle investigator
   2. Sponsor
   3. Monitor
   4. Chief investigator

   A. Appointed to verify that the study at site is in accordance with good clinical practice and the protocol, and that data collection is complete and accurate
   B. Responsible for the conduct of a study
   C. Responsible for the setup and conduct of a study in a site
   D. Ensures all legal, ethical, and financial requirements have been met. Maintains overall management responsibility for the study
c) What is a clinical trial of an investigational medicinal product (CTIMP), and who regulates such trials? *(2 marks)*
d) What are the key features of informed consent for research? *(3 marks)*

Mr Smith is a potential participant in a CTIMP trial, and Mrs Jones is a potential participant in a non-CTIMP trial. Neither have capacity to provide consent.

e) Mrs Jones's family are supportive of her participation. Do they need to sign a consent form and why/why not? *(2 marks)*
f) Mr Smith does not have any family or friends who are willing or able to provide consent. What action should the research team take? *(1 mark)*

Mrs Jones is recruited to a non-CTIMP trial after consulting her family. Mr Smith is recruited into a CTIMP trial after the professional legal representative provides consent.

g) Mrs Jones regains capacity midway through the trial. What action should the research team take with regard to ongoing participation? *(1 mark)*
h) Mr Smith also regains capacity. What action should the research team take with regard to ongoing participation? *(1 mark)*
i) What terms are used to describe each of the following occurrences? *(3 marks)*
   1. A serious untoward occurrence occurring during a study, whether related to the study or not
   2. A serious untoward occurrence caused by a study
   3. An unforeseeable serious untoward occurrence caused by the study

Answers

a) What are the potential benefits of conducting research in the NHS? *(3 marks)*

(1 mark per benefit to a maximum of 3)
- Maintains curiosity
- Promotes innovation, improved safety, and efficiency
- Encourages the discovery of new and improved treatments, investigations, and diagnoses
- Contributes to the economy
- Maintains the skills of researchers
- Empowers patients

b) Match each of the research roles to their correct description *(4 marks)*
- 1C
- 2D
- 3A
- 4B

c) What is a clinical trial of an investigational medicinal product (CTIMP), and who regulates such trials? *(2 marks)*
- Essentially any clinical trial involving medications or drugs
- They are regulated by the Medicines and Healthcare products Regulatory Agency (MHRA), who ensure that the requirements of the UK Medicines for Human Use (Clinical Trials) 2004 regulations are met

d) What are the key features of informed consent for research? *(3 marks)*
- Informed consent is a process, and as such can be withdrawn
- It is voluntary
- It is based on being given all relevant information

e) Mrs Jones's family are supportive of her participation. Do they need to sign a consent form and why/why not? *(2 marks)*
- No
- For non-CTIMP trials, a consultation process only is required

f) Mr Smith does not have any family or friends who are willing or able to provide consent. What action should the research team take? *(1 mark)*
- They should nominate an unconnected third party to act as a professional legal representative

g) Mrs Jones regains capacity midway through the trial. What action should the research team take with regard to ongoing participation? *(1 mark)*
- Mrs Jones must be asked for her consent to participate

h) Mr Smith also regains capacity. What action should the research team take with regard to ongoing participation? *(1 mark)*
- The research team would inform the patient of all elements of the study usually described in the consent process and confirm their willingness to participate. Consent has already been given by the legal representative, so it is an acceptability of ongoing participation rather than consent that is required

i) What terms are used to describe each of the following occurrences? *(3 marks)*
1. Serious adverse event
2. Serious adverse reaction
3. Serious unexpected severe adverse reaction

Notes

This question is incredibly difficult unless you're involved in research or have completed 'Good Clinical Practice' training. The link to the (free) training is provided in the 'Further reading' section, and completion of it would ensure you have the required knowledge for any questions that could be asked about the conduct of clinical research.

Further reading

National Institute for Health Research. Introduction to good clinical practice e-learning course. Available from: https://learn.nihr.ac.uk [accessed 14 February 2016].

FFICM syllabus references 11.4, 12.4, 12.15.
CoBaTrICE domains 11, 12.

OSCE 7 station 6—data

Questions

A 67-year-old HIV-positive woman has presented with a 3-week history of a dry cough and night sweats. Her chest X-ray is shown in Figure 7.4.

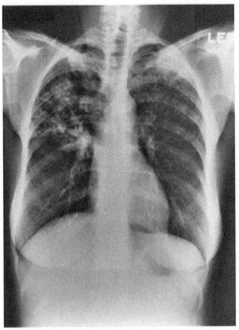

Figure 7.4 Chest X-ray

a) What is the most likely diagnosis? *(1 mark)*

b) What organisms cause tuberculosis (TB) in humans? *(1 mark)*

c) How is *Mycoplasma tuberculosis* transmitted? *(1 mark)*

d) What are the risk factors for infection with TB in European adults? *(4 marks)*

e) What antimicrobial agents should be given pending confirmation of the diagnosis of TB? *(4 marks)*

f) How many samples of sputum are required to confirm the diagnosis of active respiratory TB? *(1 mark)*

g) How and when should respiratory samples be taken? *(2 marks)*

h) What additional diagnostic test for TB disease should be performed given the patient's history of HIV infection? *(1 mark)*

i) In the context of TB, how is multidrug resistance defined? *(1 mark)*

j) How long should an inpatient with rifampicin-sensitive active pulmonary TB be cared for in a single room? *(1 mark)*

k) Which patients with active pulmonary TB should be cared for in a negative-pressure room? *(2 marks)*

l) How should latent TB be diagnosed in a patient who has previously received the Bacillus Calmette–Guérin (BCG) vaccine? *(1 mark)*

Answers

a) What is the most likely diagnosis? *(1 mark)*
   - Pulmonary tuberculosis
b) What organisms cause tuberculosis (TB) in humans? *(1 mark)*
   - *Mycoplasma tuberculosis* complex (*M. tuberculosis, M. bovis, M. africanum*)
c) How is *Mycoplasma tuberculosis* transmitted? *(1 mark)*
   - Inhalation of aerosolized sputum
d) What are the risk factors for infection with TB in European adults? *(4 marks)*

   (1 mark per risk factor to a maximum of 4)
   - HIV infection
   - Immunosuppression
   - Close contact with a person with infectious TB disease
   - Immigration from areas of the world with high rates of TB
   - Illicit drug use
   - Working or living in institutions such as hospitals, homeless shelters, prisons, nursing homes
e) What antimicrobial agents should be given pending confirmation of the diagnosis of TB?
   (4 marks)
   - Isoniazid
   - Rifampicin
   - Pyrazinamide
   - Ethambutol
f) How many samples of sputum are required to confirm the diagnosis of active respiratory TB?
   (1 mark)
   - Three
g) How and when should respiratory samples be taken? *(2 marks)*
   - Spontaneously produced, deep cough sputum samples
   - At least one should be an early morning sample
h) What additional diagnostic test for TB disease should be performed given the patient's history of HIV infection? *(1 mark)*
   - Rapid diagnostic nucleic acid amplification tests for the *M. tuberculosis* complex from the patient's sputum
i) In the context of TB, how is multidrug resistance defined? *(1 mark)*
   - Resistance to at least rifampicin and isoniazid
j) How long should an inpatient with rifampicin-sensitive active pulmonary TB be cared for in a single room? *(1 mark)*
   - At least 2 weeks since starting standard treatment
k) Which patients with active pulmonary TB should be cared for in a negative-pressure room? *(2 marks)*
   - Confirmed or suspected multidrug resistant TB
   - Patients being cared for in ward areas containing immunocompromised patients
l) How should latent TB be diagnosed in a patient who has previously received the Bacillus Calmette–Guérin (BCG) vaccine? *(1 mark)*
   - By interferon gamma release assay test (to reduce the likelihood of a false-positive result)

Further reading

Hagan G, Nathani N. Clinical review: tuberculosis on the intensive care unit. *Critical Care* 2013;17:240.
National Institute for Health and Care Excellence (NICE). Tuberculosis. NICE Guideline [NG33]. 2016. Available at: https://www.nice.org.uk/guidance/ng33 [accessed 2 May 2018].

FFICM syllabus references 2.2, 2.4, 2.6, 2.8, 3.1, 3.2, 4.2, 11.3.
CoBaTrICE domains 2, 3.

OSCE 7 station 7—data

Questions

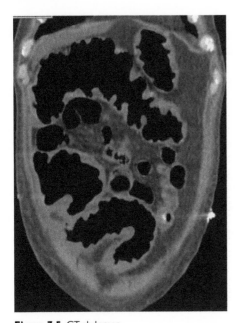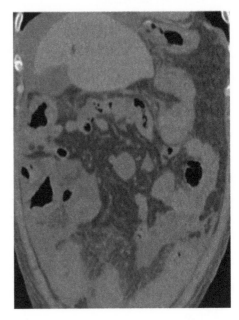

Figure 7.5 CT abdomen

Reproduced from *Gastrointestinal Imaging Cases*, Levy AD, Mortele K, and Yeh, BM, Case 64. © 2013 Oxford University Press. Reproduced with permission of the Licensor through PLSclear

You have been asked to review a patient with neutropenic sepsis following chemotherapy for acute myeloid leukaemia. The patient had been absorbing nasogastric feed with normal bowel motions, but over the last 12 hours he has developed diarrhoea, vomiting, abdominal pain, and distension. His abdomen is diffusely tender with scant bowel sounds and is tympanic to percussion.

Look at Figure 7.5.

a) What abnormalities are present on these computed tomography (CT) images? *(4 marks)*

b) What processes in the bowel wall result in the 'thumbprint' sign on imaging? *(1 mark)*

c) What are the commonest causes of the 'thumbprint' sign? *(2 marks)*

d) Which areas of the bowel are typically affected in neutropenic colitis? *(2 marks)*

Stool culture identifies the presence of *Clostridium difficile* toxin.

e) What features indicate severe (fulminant) *Clostridium difficile* infection (CDI)? *(4 marks)*

f) What are the first-line treatment options for severe CDI? *(2 marks)*

g) What are the treatment options for resistant severe CDI? *(5 marks)*

Answers

a) What abnormalities are present on these computed tomography (CT) images? *(4 marks)*
   - Dilated gas-filled colon
   - Colonic wall thickening with thumbprinting and pseudo-polyp formation
   - Intra-abdominal free fluid
   - Pericolic fat stranding

b) What processes in the bowel wall result in the 'thumbprint' sign on imaging? *(1 mark)*
   - Oedema or haemorrhage

c) What are the commonest causes of the 'thumbprint' sign? *(2 marks)*

   (1 mark per cause to a maximum of 2)
   - Infective colitis
   - Ischaemic colitis
   - Inflammatory bowel disease

d) Which areas of the bowel are typically affected in neutropenic colitis? *(2 marks)*
   - Ileo-caecum
   - Ascending colon

e) What features indicate severe (fulminant) *Clostridium difficile* infection (CDI)? *(4 marks)*

   (1 mark per feature to a maximum of 4)
   - Leucocytosis—white cell count >15 × 10^9/L
   - Acute kidney injury with a creatinine rise of >50% of baseline or >133 µmol/L
   - Temperature >38.5°C
   - Hypotension or shock
   - Clinical evidence of severe colitis
   - Radiological evidence of severe colitis

f) What are the first-line treatment options for severe CDI? *(2 marks)*
   - Enteral vancomycin for 10–14 days
   - Fidaxomicin in those at high risk for recurrence, e.g. the elderly and those receiving antibiotics

g) What are the treatment options for resistant severe CDI? *(5 marks)*

   (1 mark per treatment to a maximum of 5)
   - High-dose enteral vancomycin
   - Intravenous (IV) metronidazole
   - Oral fidaxomicin
   - Colonic vancomycin
   - IV immunoglobulin
   - Faecal transplant
   - Surgery

Further reading

James B, Kelly B. The abdominal radiograph. *Ulster Medical Journal* 2013;82:179–187.

McDonald LC, Gerding DN, Johnson S, Bakken JS, Carroll KC, Coffin SE, et al. Clinical practice guidelines for Clostridium difficile infection in adults and children: 2017 Update by the Infectious Diseases Society of America (IDSA) and Society for Healthcare Epidemiology of America (SHEA). *Clinical Infectious Diseases* 2018;66:e1–e48.

Wilcox MH. *Updated Guidance on the Management and Treatment of Clostridium difficile Infection*. PHE gateway number: 2013043. London: Public Health England. 2013.

FFICM syllabus references 2.2, 2.4, 2.6, 3.1, 3.7, 4.1, 4.2.
CoBaTrICE domains 2, 3, 4.

OSCE 7 station 8—data

Questions

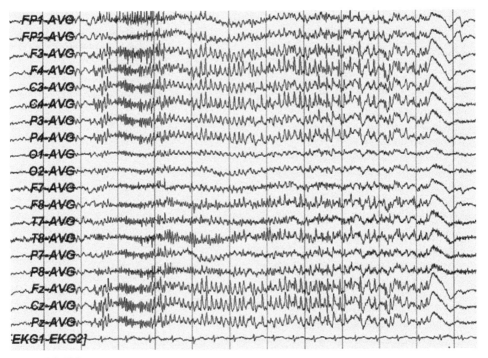

Figure 7.6 EEG

Reproduced from *Atlas of EEG, Seizure Seminology, and Management*, Misulis KE, Figure 4.140. © 2013 Oxford University Press, Reproduced with permission of the Licensor through PLSclear

A 55-year-old man was admitted to the critical care unit having been intubated and ventilated in the emergency department for treatment of a seizure lasting >2 hours. Lorazepam, levetiracetam, and phenytoin had been ineffective in terminating the seizure. An electroencephalogram (EEG) was recorded on day 3, while sedated with thiopentone, midazolam, and fentanyl.

Look at Figure 7.6.

a) What does the EEG show? *(1 mark)*
b) What are the potential sources of EEG artefact in the critical care unit? *(3 marks)*
c) What is the diagnosis? *(1 mark)*
d) What atypical pharmacological agents have been used to terminate seizures in refractory status epilepticus? *(3 marks)*

Despite stopping sedation on day 5, the patient's Glasgow Coma Scale score on day 9 remained as E1, V1, M1. There was no evidence of further seizures, and pupillary responses were normal. A computed tomography scan of the head showed global loss of grey–white differentiation and effacement of the ventricles.

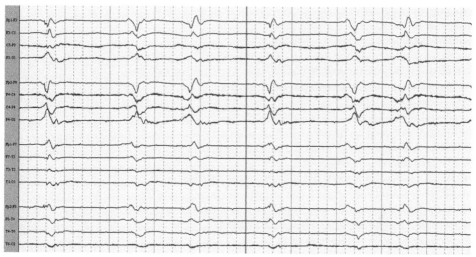

Figure 7.7 EEG

Reproduced from *Atlas of EEG, Seizure Seminology, and Management*, Misulis KE, Figure 4.83. © 2013 Oxford University Press, Reproduced with permission of the Licensor through PLSclear

Look at Figure 7.7.

e) Describe the EEG *(2 marks)*

f) What is the most likely cause of these EEG findings? *(1 mark)*

Somatosensory evoked potentials were performed to aid prognostication.

g) How are somatosensory evoked potentials performed? *(4 marks)*

h) What effect do neuromuscular drugs have on somatosensory evoked potentials? *(1 mark)*

i) What other types of evoked potential are in clinical use, and when might they be used? *(4 marks)*

Answers

a) What does the EEG show? *(1 mark)*
  - Waveforms of variable frequency and amplitude typical of seizure activity
b) What are the potential sources of EEG artefact in the critical care unit? *(3 marks)*
  - Muscle activity, e.g. shivering, ocular movement
  - Therapy, e.g. mouth care, suctioning, extracorporeal circuits such as renal replacement therapy
  - Equipment, e.g. interference from pressure regulating or percussive mattress, ventilators, IV infusion devices
c) What is the diagnosis? *(1 mark)*
  - Refractory status epilepticus
d) What atypical pharmacological agents have been used to terminate seizures in refractory status epilepticus? *(3 marks)*

Atypical agents are drugs that are not primarily known for their anticonvulsive properties and that are not in standard status epilepticus management protocols.
  (1 mark per agent to a maximum of 3)
  - Ketamine
  - Magnesium
  - Inhaled anaesthetic agents—e.g. isoflurane, desflurane
  - Immunomodulation—corticosteroids, immunosuppression, immunoglobulin
  - Intravenous ketogenic diet
e) Describe the EEG *(2 marks)*
  - Baseline 'suppression' (flattened isoelectric base line)
  - Infrequent 'bursts' of variable low amplitude spikes
f) What is the most likely cause of these EEG findings? *(1 mark)*
  - Hypoxic ischaemic brain injury (also known as hypoxic encephalopathy)
g) How are somatosensory evoked potentials performed? *(4 marks)*
  - An electrical stimulus is delivered to a peripheral nerve (commonly the median or tibial nerve)
  - Cortical scalp electrodes are positioned over the sensory area of the cortex corresponding to the nerve being studied
  - A 'ground' skin electrode placed between the stimulus and the cortical receiving device to confirm that electrical transmission has occurred via an intact nerve to the spinal cord
  - A cortical EEG is recorded, and the latency and amplitude of the averaged cortical waveform are compared to healthy norms
h) What effect do neuromuscular drugs have on somatosensory evoked potentials? *(1 mark)*
  - No effect, because it is the sensory rather than motor pathway that is being studied
i) What other types of evoked potential are in clinical use, and when might they be used? *(4 marks)*

  (2 marks for each example of an evoked potential modality with a correct clinical application)
  - Brainstem auditory:
    - Diagnosis, e.g. demyelinating disease or brainstem lesions
    - Perioperative monitoring, e.g. acoustic neuroma surgery
  - Visual:
    - Diagnosis and monitoring of pathology causing optic neuritis and ischaemia
    - Perioperative monitoring, e.g. pituitary surgery
  - Somatosensory and motor:
    - Perioperative, e.g. scoliosis surgery, open descending thoracic aortic surgery

Further reading

Danayach NS, Claassen J. Electrophysiology in the intensive care unit. In: Smith MM, Citerio GG, Kofke AJ (eds.) *Oxford Textbook of Neurocritical Care*, pp. 161–180. Oxford: Oxford University Press; 2016.

Shorvon S, Ferlisi M. The treatment of super-refractory status epilepticus: a critical review of available therapies and a clinical treatment protocol. *Brain* 2011;134;2802–2818.

FFICM syllabus references 1.1, 2.6, 3.1, 3.6.
CoBaTrICE domains 2, 3.

OSCE 7 station 9—data

Questions

One of your patients has just returned from the computed tomography (CT) scanner. The radiologist tells you that 'There is a lesion in the parietotemporal area. It is thick walled and round. It has a central area of low attenuation and the wall is enhancing with contrast'.

a) What is the differential diagnosis for a cerebral ring-enhancing lesion? *(5 marks)*

b) What are the three most common presenting symptoms of a solitary brain abscess? *(3 marks)*

c) Other than the abscess itself, what other intracerebral abnormalities might be seen on CT in a patient with this pathology? *(3 marks)*

d) What are the potential causes of a brain abscess? *(4 marks)*

e) In which lobes of the brain are abscesses most common? *(2 marks)*

f) What features of a brain abscess make a favourable outcome unlikely? *(3 marks)*

Answers

a) What is the differential diagnosis for a cerebral ring-enhancing lesion? *(5 marks)*

(1 mark per diagnosis to a maximum of 5)
- Brain abscess
- Malignancy—metastasis, glioblastoma, cerebral lymphoma
- Treatment related—postoperative change or radiation necrosis
- Resolving haematoma or cerebral contusion
- Subacute infarct
- Tuberculoma
- Demyelinating disease

b) What are the three most common presenting symptoms of a solitary brain abscess? *(3 marks)*
- Headache
- Focal neurological deficit
- Fever

c) Other than the abscess itself, what other intracerebral abnormalities might be seen on CT in a patient with this pathology? *(3 marks)*
- Surrounding areas of low attenuation (oedema)
- Contrast enhancement of the ventricular wall (ventriculitis)
- Mass effect

d) What are the potential causes of a brain abscess? *(4 marks)*
- Local infection—dental infection, mastoiditis, otitis media, sinusitis
- Septic emboli
- Haematogenous spread from distant infection (e.g. pneumonia)
- Direct inoculation (traumatic foreign body or operative infection)

e) In which lobes of the brain are abscesses most common? *(2 marks)*
- Frontal
- Temporal

f) What features of a bacterial brain abscess make a favourable outcome unlikely? *(3 marks)*

- Ventricular rupture
- Decreased level of consciousness before antibiotic therapy
- Rapid symptom onset

Further reading

Wijdicks E. Brain abscesses. In: *The Practice of Emergency and Critical Care Neurology*, 2nd Edition, pp. 460–473. Oxford: Oxford University Press; 2016.

FFICM syllabus references 2.2, 2.6, 3.1, 3.6, 3.9.
CoBaTrICE domains 2, 3.

OSCE 7 station 10—data

Questions

a) What are the disadvantages of using conventional laboratory-based tests of coagulation in the bleeding patient? *(4 marks)*

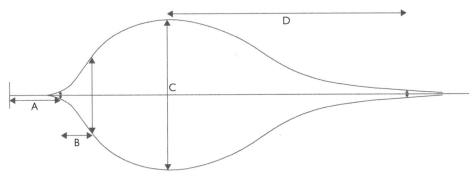

Figure 7.8 Viscoelastic haemostatic assay

Figure 7.8 shows a trace of a viscoelastic haemostatic assay (VHA).

b) Complete Table 7.2q to identify the labelled parameters *(7 marks)*

Table 7.2q VHA parameters

Parameter	Terminology used in the TEG® system	Terminology used in the ROTEM® system
A		
B		
C		
D		N/A

c) What is the amplitude of the trace at the beginning and the end of time period B? *(2 marks)*
d) What is the amplitude of the trace at the end of time period D? *(1 mark)*
e) What does the alpha angle measure? *(1 mark)*

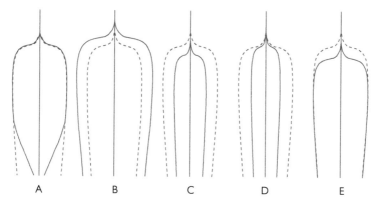

A   B   C   D   E

Figure 7.9 Abnormal viscoelastic haemostatic assays

Look at Figure 7.9.

f) Which VHA trace would be seen in each of the following clinical scenarios (the dashed line represents a normal trace)? *(5 marks)*
- Clotting factor deficiency
- Hypercoagulable state
- Global hypocoagulable state
- Hyperfibrinolysis
- Thrombocytopenia

Answers

a) What are the disadvantages of using conventional laboratory-based tests of coagulation in the bleeding patient? *(4 marks)*
   - Long turnaround time (results may no longer be clinically accurate in a dynamic situation)
   - Laboratory-based tests are poor predictors of bleeding risk
   - Laboratory-based tests are poor predictors of blood product usage
   - Conventional laboratory tests do not examine the entire process of coagulation

b) Complete Table 7.2a to identify the labelled parameters *(7 marks)*

Table 7.2a VHA parameters

Parameter	Terminology used in the TEG® system	Terminology used in the ROTEM® system
A	R time	Clot time
B	K time	Clot formation time
C	Maximum amplitude	Maximum clot firmness
D	Clot lysis time	N/A

c) What is the amplitude of the trace at the beginning and the end of time period B? *(2 marks)*
   - 2 mm at the beginning
   - 20 mm at the end

d) What is the amplitude of the trace at the end of time period D? *(1 mark)*
   - 2 mm

e) What does the alpha angle measure? *(1 mark)*
   - The rate of clot formation

f) Which VHA trace would be seen in each of the following clinical scenarios (the dashed line represents a normal trace)? *(5 marks)*
   - Clotting factor deficiency—E
   - Hypercoagulable state—B
   - Global hypocoagulable state—C
   - Hyperfibrinolysis—A
   - Thrombocytopenia—D

Notes

Unfortunately, there are some topics that simply need to be memorized for the exam (such as the terminology in this question). This is also the type of question that can really knock your confidence if you are unfamiliar with the subject, but if you keep your head and take your time you will score marks for the sections that can be answered with a bit of 'on the spot working out' or educated guesswork!

Further reading

Mallett SV, Cox D. Thrombelastography. *British Journal of Anaesthesia* 1992;69:307–313.

FFICM syllabus references 1.5, 2.2, 2.8, 4.3, 6.1.
CoBaTrICE domains 1, 2.

OSCE 7 station 11—data

Questions

A 60-year-old man is admitted to the intensive care unit. His liver function tests are as follows (normal ranges in brackets):

- Bilirubin 84 μmol/L (3–17 μmol/L)
- Alanine aminotransferase (ALT) 123 U/L (5–35 U/L)
- Aspartate aminotransferase (AST) 78 U/L (5–35 U/L)
- Alkaline phosphatase (ALP) 578 U/L (30–130 U/L)
- Gamma-glutamyl transferase (GGT) 167 U/L (11–51 U/L)

a) Which tissues, other than the liver, contain ALT? *(3 marks)*

b) What pathophysiological process is the most likely cause of these liver function tests? *(1 mark)*

c) What imaging investigation would you request? *(1 mark)*

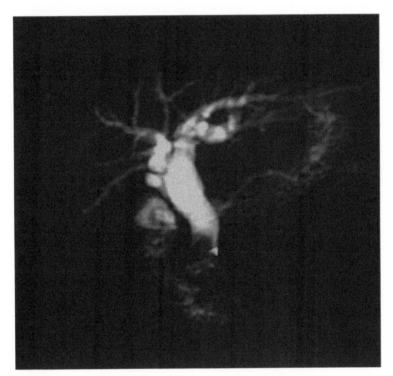

Figure 7.10 MRCP

Reproduced from *Emergencies in Clinical Radiology*, Graham R and Gallagher F, Figure 7.10. © 2009 Oxford University Press. Reproduced with permission of the Licensor through PLSclear

An ultrasound examination reveals an enlarged (12 × 6 cm), thick-walled gallbladder with visible sludge and a poorly visualized common bile duct. Magnetic resonance cholangiopancreatography (MRCP) was performed (Figure 7.10).

d) What abnormal findings are seen on the MRCP? *(2 marks)*

An endoscopic retrograde cholangiopancreatogram (ERCP) was performed to remove the common bile duct stone.

e) What are the potential complications of ERCP? *(5 marks)*

f) What class of medication has been shown to be useful in the prevention of post-ERCP pancreatitis? *(1 mark)*

A second patient develops the following abnormal liver function tests 5 days after starting treatment with phenytoin (normal ranges in brackets):

- Bilirubin 31 µmol/L (3–17 µmol/L)
- ALT 1027 U/L (5–35 U/L)
- AST 786 U/L (5–35 U/L)
- ALP 194 U/L (30–130 U/L)
- GGT 87 U/L (11–51 U/L)

g) How can liver function tests help determine whether a drug has caused a cholecystatic or hepatocellular injury? *(2 marks)*

h) What is the significance of a raised serum bilirubin level in cases of drug-induced hepatocellular injury? *(1 mark)*

i) How might phenytoin affect the plasma concentrations of other hepatically metabolized drugs, and why? *(2 marks)*

j) How might nasogastric feed affect the plasma concentration of phenytoin, and why? *(2 marks)*

Answers

a) Which tissues, other than the liver, contain ALT *(3 marks)*
- Heart
- Skeletal muscle
- Kidney

b) What pathophysiological process is the most likely cause of these liver function tests? *(1 mark)*
- Biliary obstruction

c) What imaging investigation would you request? *(1 mark)*
- Abdominal ultrasound

d) What abnormal findings are seen on the MRCP? *(2 marks)*
- Dilated biliary tree
- Obstructing calculus in the distal common bile duct

e) What are the potential complications of ERCP? *(5 marks)*
- Perforation
- Haemorrhage
- Pancreatitis
- Infection (usually cholangitis)
- Stent-related complications (e.g. occlusion, misplacement, migration)

f) What class of medication has been shown to be useful in the prevention of post-ERCP pancreatitis? *(1 mark)*
- Non-steroidal anti-inflammatory drugs

g) How can liver function tests help determine whether a drug has caused a cholecystatic or hepatocellular injury? *(2 marks)*
- ALP >2× upper limit of normal and an ALT/ALP ratio <2 suggests a cholecystatic injury
- ALT >3× upper limit of normal and an ALT/ALP ratio >5 suggests a hepatocellular injury

h) What is the significance of a raised serum bilirubin level in cases of drug-induced hepatocellular injury? *(1 mark)*
- A raised serum bilirubin level is associated with increased mortality (Hys law)

i) How might phenytoin affect the plasma concentrations of other hepatically metabolized drugs, and why? *(2 marks)*
- Phenytoin can cause a reduction in the plasma concentrations of such drugs …
- … because phenytoin is a potent inducer of cytochrome p450 enzymes

j) How might nasogastric feed affect the plasma concentration of phenytoin, and why? *(2 marks)*
- Nasogastric feed can cause a reduced plasma phenytoin concentration …
- … because of reduced gastric absorption of phenytoin

Notes

This question covers a lot of ground but asks very direct questions. If you're asked a direct question to which you don't know the answer you should guess or just tell the examiner you don't know—either way you don't want to lose time when you could be picking up marks on later bits of the question. Because of the way the questions are written, not knowing one answer won't jeopardize you later.

Further reading

Devarbhavi H. An update on drug-induced liver injury. *Journal of Clinical and Experimental Hepatology* 2012;2:247–259.
European Association for the Study of the Liver. EASL Clinical Practice Guidelines: Management of cholestatic liver diseases. *Journal of Hepatology* 2009;51:237–267.

FFICM syllabus references 2.2, 2.6, 2.8, 3.7, 4.1.
CoBaTrICE domains 2, 4.

OSCE 7 station 12—equipment

Questions

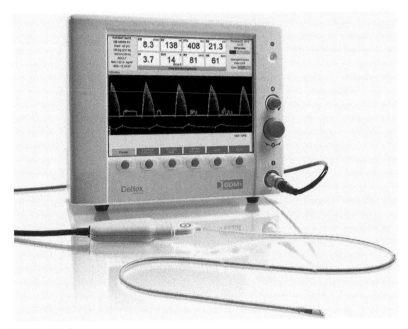

Figure 7.11 Medical device
Reproduced with kind permission from Deltex Medical

Look at Figure 7.11.

a) What is this piece of equipment? *(1 mark)*
b) What does the oesophageal Doppler probe measure? *(1 mark)*
c) What would be a typical depth of insertion via the nose and mouth? *(2 marks)*
d) What patient-specific information does the oesophageal Doppler monitor use to estimate the cross-sectional area of the aorta? *(3 marks)*
e) What assumptions are made when deriving data from the oesophageal Doppler? *(4 marks)*

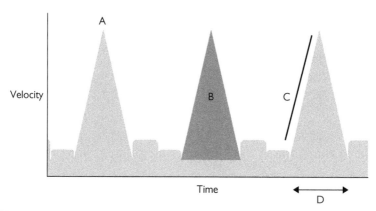

Figure 7.12 Oesophageal Doppler waveform

Look at the normal oesophageal Doppler waveform in Figure 7.12.

f) Define the parameters A–D *(4 marks)*
g) The stroke distance (area B) correlates with which physiological variable? *(1 mark)*
h) The flow time (distance D) is inversely related to which determinants of cardiac output? *(2 marks)*
i) The peak velocity (parameter A) correlates with which determinant of cardiac output? *(1 mark)*

Answers

a) What is this piece of equipment? *(1 mark)*
  - Oesophageal Doppler cardiac output monitor
b) What does the oesophageal Doppler probe measure? *(1 mark)*
  - The velocity of blood flow in the descending aorta
c) What would be a typical depth of insertion via the nose and mouth? *(2 marks)*
  - Oral—35 to 40 cm
  - Nasal—40 to 45 cm
d) What patient-specific information does the oesophageal Doppler monitor use to estimate the cross-sectional area of the aorta? *(3 marks)*
  - Age
  - Height
  - Weight
e) What assumptions are made when deriving data from the oesophageal Doppler? *(4 marks)*

  (1 mark per assumption to a maximum of 4)
  - The probe placement is optimal
  - The aorta is a uniform cylinder
  - The ratio of ascending to descending aortic flow is fixed
  - The nomogram accurately calculates true aortic cross-sectional area
  - There is no diastolic aortic blood flow
f) Define the parameters A–D *(4 marks)*
  A—peak velocity
  B—stroke distance
  C—mean acceleration
  D—flow time
g) The stroke distance (area B) correlates with which physiological variable? *(1 mark)*
  - Stroke volume
h) The flow time (distance D) is inversely related to which determinants of cardiac output? *(2 marks)*
  - Heart rate
  - Afterload
i) The peak velocity (parameter A) correlates with which determinant of cardiac output? *(1 mark)*
  - Contractility

Notes

If you don't come from an anaesthesia background this question is likely to be unfamiliar. The oesophageal Doppler is specifically named in the UK syllabus so we have included it as a reminder to be familiar with it, at least in theory. All you could realistically be asked about it is covered in this question.

Further reading

Singer M. Oesophageal Doppler. *Current Opinion in Critical Care* 2009;15:244–248.

FFICM syllabus references 2.7, 5.14.
CoBaTrICE domain 2.

OSCE 7 station 13—equipment

Questions

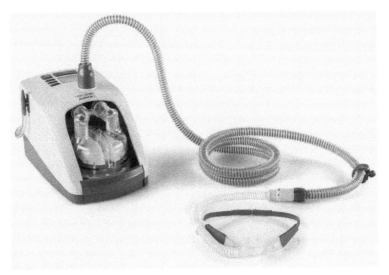

Figure 7.13 Medical device
Reproduced with kind permission from Fisher and Paykel

You are asked to review a 59-year-old man on the respiratory ward with pneumonia. He was admitted 24 hours ago and has become increasingly hypoxaemic. The outreach team have begun therapy with the equipment shown in Figure 7.13.

a) What is this piece of equipment? *(1 mark)*

b) What are the features of high-flow nasal oxygen (HFNO) that help in hypoxic respiratory failure? *(3 marks)*

c) Other than hypoxic respiratory failure, what other uses are there for HFNO? *(5 marks)*

The patient is taken to intensive care and intubated. The following day it is suggested he undergoes a spontaneous breathing trial (SBT) with a view to extubation

d) What factors should be assessed to judge whether a patient is suitable for extubation? *(5 marks)*

e) What steps are involved in conducting a SBT? *(3 marks)*

f) How is the rapid shallow breathing index (RSBI) calculated? *(1 mark)*

g) How can the RSBI be used to assess readiness for extubation? *(2 marks)*

Answers

a) What is this piece of equipment? *(1 mark)*
   - High-flow nasal oxygen device
b) What are the features of high-flow nasal oxygen (HFNO) delivery that help in hypoxic respiratory failure? *(3 marks)*
   - Humidification
   - High FiO_2
   - Continuous positive airway pressure effect
c) Other than hypoxic respiratory failure, what other uses are there for HFNO in adults? *(5 marks)*
   - Intubation (pre-oxygenation and apnoeic oxygenation)
   - Post-extubation respiratory distress
   - Palliative symptom relief
   - Prevention of respiratory failure post cardiac surgery
   - Oxygen supply during procedures where sedation is used and access to the mouth is required, e.g. bronchoscopy, trans-oesophageal echocardiography, and endoscopy
d) What factors should be assessed to judge whether a patient is suitable for extubation? *(5 marks)*

   (1 mark per answer to a maximum of 5)
   - Lung pathology is stable or resolving
   - Spontaneous cough with manageable secretion load
   - Low oxygen (e.g. <50%) and positive end-expiratory pressure (PEEP) (e.g. <5–8 cmH$_2$O) requirement
   - Haemodynamic stability
   - Able to initiate and maintain sufficient spontaneous breaths
   - Alert and not distressed
   - Pain is controlled
e) What steps are involved in conducting a SBT? *(3 marks)*
   - The patient is allowed to breathe spontaneously. If attached to a ventilator, 'minimal ventilator settings' are used (e.g. pressure support of 5–7 cmH$_2$O and 1–5 cmH$_2$O PEEP)
   - The trial should last 30–120 minutes
   - Objective measures are made of patient comfort and respiratory function
f) How is the rapid shallow breathing index (RSBI) calculated? *(1 mark)*
   - Respiratory rate divided by tidal volume (in litres)
g) How can the RSBI be used to assess readiness for extubation? *(2 marks)*

   - An RSBI of <105 suggests an 80% chance of successful extubation
   - An RSBI of >105 strongly suggests weaning failure

Further reading

Ashraf-Kashani N, Kumar R. High-flow nasal oxygen therapy. *BJA Education* 2017:17:57–62.

Esteban A, Frutos F, Tobin MJ, Alía I, Solsona JF, Valverdú I, et al. A comparison of four methods of weaning patients from mechanical ventilation. Spanish Lung Failure Collaborative Group. *New England Journal of Medicine* 1995;332:345–350.

FFICM syllabus references 3.1, 3.8, 4.6, 5.1.
CoBaTrICE domains 1, 4, 6.

OSCE 8

OSCE 8 station 1—professionalism

Questions

It is 2 am, and one of your colleagues tells you that they have 'pricked their finger' while stitching in a central line on the high dependency unit. Your colleague shows you a bleeding puncture mark and asks the following questions:

a) 'What do I need to do about the wound?' (2 marks)
b) 'What else needs to be done?' (5 marks)
c) 'Does this all need to be done tonight?' (1 mark)
d) 'What bloods need to be taken from the patient?' (3 marks)
e) 'What happens to the blood sample taken from me tonight?' (1 mark)
f) 'Is there anything I can do to avoid getting another sharps injury in the future?' (5 marks)

Answers

a) 'What do I need to do about the wound?' *(2 marks)*
- Wash the wound with soap and water
- Encourage free bleeding

b) 'What else needs to be done?' *(5 marks)*
- A risk assessment of the patient must be carried out by another member of the team
- The donor patient will have bloods taken after providing consent
- The injured colleague needs to attend the emergency department (or another nominated clinical area) with the completed risk assessment
- The injured colleague will have a blood sample taken and their hepatitis B immunization status established
- An incident form must be completed

c) 'Does this all need to be done tonight?' *(1 mark)*
- Yes, if post-exposure prophylaxis is required it should be started as soon as possible post injury

d) 'What blood tests need to be taken from the patient?' *(3 marks)*
- HIV antibodies
- Hepatitis B surface antigen
- Hepatitis C antibodies

e) 'What happens to the blood sample taken from me tonight?' *(1 mark)*
- It is stored, and tested only if subsequent blood samples are positive

f) 'Is there anything I can do to avoid getting another sharps injury in the future?' *(5 marks)*

(1 mark per suggestion to a maximum of 5)
- Avoid using sharps where possible or use a sharp safe alternative if available
- Plan for safe disposal of sharps before use, and avoid leaving sharps lying around
- Don't re-sheath needles
- Don't bend or break needles
- Place used sharps in an approved sharps bin placed immediately next to you
- Don't overfill sharps containers
- Don't try to remove items from a sharps container
- Keep up to date with and uphold relevant local policies and procedures

General communication *(3 marks)*

Marks awarded for behaviours such as the following:
- Pace and volume of speech
- Demonstrates empathy and addresses concerns
- Offers clear explanations

Further reading

Local sharps/needlestick policy.

FFICM syllabus references 11.2, 11.3, 11.4, 12.2.
CoBaTrICE domain 11.

OSCE 8 station 2—resuscitation

Questions

You are called to an adult patient in cardiac arrest. The nursing staff are providing cardiopulmonary resuscitation (CPR).

a) What are your first actions? *(4 marks)*

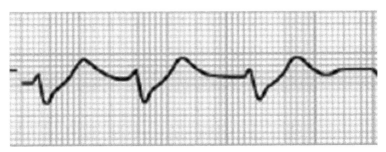

Figure 8.1 Rhythm strip

Reproduced from *Oxford Handbook of Clinical Medicine, Tenth Edition*, Wilkinson IB, Raine T, and Wiles K, Figure 14.4. © 2017 Oxford University Press. Reproduced with permission of the Licensor through PLSclear

You confirm cardiorespiratory arrest and are given a printout of the rhythm strip from the defibrillator. Look at Figure 8.1.

b) How would you describe the morphology of the electrocardiogram? *(2 marks)*

c) Which Resuscitation Council (UK) advanced life support algorithm should you follow? *(1 mark)*

d) How would you proceed in the setting of a cardiac arrest with pulseless electrical activity? *(6 marks)*

e) What is the recommended rate of chest compressions in the Resuscitation Council (UK) guidelines? *(1 mark)*

f) What is the recommended depth of chest compressions in the Resuscitation Council (UK) guidelines? *(1 mark)*

At the end of 2 minutes the patient has no pulse and the monitored rhythm is unchanged.

g) How you would proceed? *(2 marks)*

You discover the patient has a potassium level of 8.4 mmol/L (normal range: 3.5–5 mmol/L)

h) What medications are recommended during cardiac arrest in the presence of hyperkalaemia? *(3 marks)*

Answers

a) What are your first actions? *(4 marks)*
- Confirm cardiorespiratory arrest
- Call the cardiac arrest team
- Continue CPR at a ratio of 30 cardiac compressions to 2 ventilation breaths with supplementary oxygen
- Attach a defibrillator to assess the cardiac rhythm

b) How would you describe the morphology of the electrocardiogram? *(2 marks)*
- Sine wave
- Broad QRS with absent P waves

c) Which Resuscitation Council (UK) advanced life support algorithm should you follow? *(1 mark)*
- Non-shockable rhythms—pulseless electrical activity

d) How would you proceed in the setting of a cardiac arrest with pulseless electrical activity? *(6 marks)*
- Ensure the airway is patent, using airway adjuncts, supraglottic airway devices, and intubation as required
- Continue good-quality CPR with minimal interruptions
- Attach capnography
- Establish vascular access
- Administer 1 mg adrenaline followed by a saline flush
- Evaluate and treat the reversible causes of cardiac arrest

e) What is the recommended rate of chest compressions in the Resuscitation Council (UK) guidelines? *(1 mark)*
- 100–120 compressions/minute

f) What is the recommended depth of chest compressions in the Resuscitation Council (UK) guidelines? *(1 mark)*
- 5–6 cm or ⅓ of the depth of the chest

g) How you would proceed? *(2 marks)*
- Promptly restart CPR at a ratio of 30 cardiac compressions to 2 ventilation breaths with supplementary oxygen
- Continue CPR for a further 2 minutes with minimal interruptions

h) What medications are recommended during cardiac arrest in the presence of hyperkalaemia? *(3 marks)*
- Calcium chloride
- Sodium bicarbonate
- Insulin and dextrose

Notes

This question should be straightforward, but in an exam setting nothing can be taken for granted. If possible, find a mannequin and practise the life support algorithms in advance.

Further reading

Resuscitation Council (UK). Adult advanced life support. 2015. Available at: https://www.resus.org.uk/resuscitation-guidelines/adult-advanced-life-support/ [accessed 11 June 2018].

FFICM syllabus references 1.1, 1.2, 2.3, 4.8, 5.1, 11.6.
CoBaTrICE domains 1, 2.

OSCE 8 station 3—data

Questions

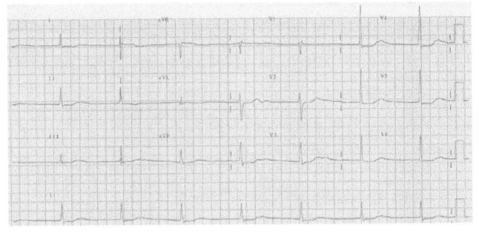

Figure 8.2 Electrocardiogram (ECG)

Reproduced from *Emergencies in Cardiology, Second Edition*, Myerson SG et al., Figure 21.38. © 2009 Oxford University Press. Reproduced with permission of the Licensor through PLSclear

You are asked to see a 63-year-old man who has lost consciousness several times following an elective parathyroidectomy. The patient's electrocardiogram (ECG) is shown in Figure 8.2.

a) What abnormalities are present on this ECG? *(4 marks)*

b) In which lead should the QT interval be measured *(1 mark)*

c) Where is the QT interval measured? *(2 marks)*

d) What is the relationship between changes in the heart rate and the QT interval? *(1 mark)*

e) State Bazett's formula *(1 mark)*

f) What electrolyte abnormalities are commonly associated with a prolonged QT interval? *(3 marks)*

The serum calcium concentration is 1.5 mmol//L (2.12–2.60) and serum magnesium 0.43 mmol/L (0.75–1.05).

g) How should the measured calcium concentration be corrected for changes in the concentration of serum albumin? *(1 mark)*

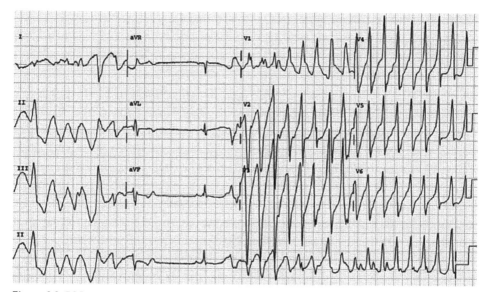

Figure 8.3 ECG

Reproduced from *Heart Disease in Pregnancy*, Adamson DL, Dhanjal MK, and Nelson-Piercy C, Figure 9.5. © 2011 Oxford University Press. Reproduced with permission of the Licensor through PLSclear

The patient suddenly becomes more unwell, with a blood pressure of 76/53 mmHg. He is clammy and confused. You notice his ECG has suddenly changed.

Look at Figure 8.3.

h) What is the diagnosis? *(1 mark)*

i) What treatment is urgently required? *(1 mark)*

Sinus rhythm is restored and electrolyte infusions are commenced.

j) Other than correction of electrolyte abnormalities, what other treatment options are available to prevent the ventricular tachycardia recurring? *(3 marks)*

k) Which classes of antiarrhythmic drugs should be avoided in this patient? *(2 marks)*

Answers

a) What abnormalities are present on this ECG? *(4 marks)*
  - Bradycardia
  - Prolonged QT interval
  - P waves not visible
  - 1 mm ST depression in I, V4–6

b) In which lead should the QT interval be measured *(1 mark)*
  - II

c) Where is the QT interval measured? *(2 marks)*
  - From the beginning of the QRS complex ...
  - ... to the end of the T wave

d) What is the relationship between changes in the heart rate and the QT interval? *(1 mark)*
  - Inverse relationship

e) State Bazett's formula *(1 mark)*
  - Corrected QT interval = measured QT interval/√ RR interval

f) What electrolyte abnormalities are commonly associated with a prolonged QT interval? *(3 marks)*
  - Hypocalcaemia
  - Hypomagnesaemia
  - Hypokalaemia

g) How should the measured calcium concentration be corrected for changes in the concentration of serum albumin? *(1 mark)*
  - Corrected calcium = measured calcium + 0.02 × (40 – [albumin] (g/L))

h) What is the diagnosis? *(1 mark)*
  - Polymorphic ventricular tachycardia (torsades de pointes)

i) What treatment is urgently required? *(1 mark)*
  - Synchronized direct current (DC) cardioversion

j) Other than correction of electrolyte abnormalities, what other treatment options are available to prevent the ventricular tachycardia recurring? *(3 marks)*
  - Stopping medications that could prolong the QT interval
  - Increasing the heart rate using medication
  - Electrical pacing

k) Which classes of antiarrhythmic drugs should be avoided in this patient? *(2 marks)*
  - Class I
  - Class III

Further reading

Beed M, Sherman R, Mahajan R. Metabolic, endocrine, and environmental injury. In: Beed M, Sherman R, Mahajan R (eds.) *Emergencies in Critical Care*, 2nd Edition, pp. 203–254. Oxford: Oxford University Press; 2013.

Murray S. ECG recognition. In: Myerson S, Choudhury R, Mitchell A (eds.) *Emergencies in Cardiology*, 2nd Edition, pp. 383–430. Oxford: Oxford University Press; 2010.

Postema PG, Wilde AAM. The measurement of the QT interval. *Current Cardiology Reviews* 2014;10: 287–294.

FFICM syllabus references 1.1, 1.2, 2.2, 2.3, 2.7, 2.8, 3.1, 3.3, 4.1, 4.4, 4.8.
CoBaTrICE domains 1, 2, 3.

OSCE 8 station 4—data

Questions

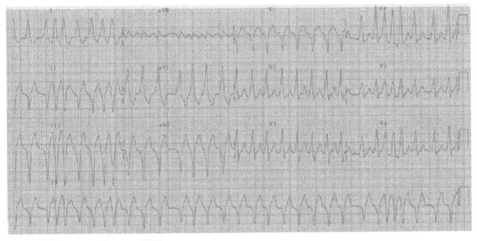

Figure 8.4 Electrocardiogram (ECG)

Reproduced from *Emergencies in Cardiology, Second Edition*, Myerson SG et al., Figure 21.29. © 2009 Oxford University Press. Reproduced with permission of the Licensor through PLSclear

Look at the electrocardiogram (ECG) in Figure 8.4.

a) Describe this ECG *(6 marks)*
b) What is the diagnosis? *(1 mark)*
c) What ECG features suggest that a broad complex tachycardia is ventricular in origin? *(5 marks)*
d) What is the definition of pre-excitation? *(2 marks)*
e) Describe the potential resting ECG findings seen in a patient with an accessory pathway *(2 marks)*
f) What pharmacological agents are used for the treatment of atrial fibrillation with pre-excitation in the haemodynamically stable patient? *(2 marks)*
g) What is the treatment for atrial fibrillation with pre-excitation in the haemodynamically unstable patient? *(1 mark)*
h) Define the Wolff–Parkinson–White syndrome *(1 mark)*

Answers

a) Describe this ECG *(6 marks)*
- Irregular rhythm
- Rate 150–300 beats per minute
- No visible P waves
- Broad QRS of variable duration
- Left axis deviation
- T-wave inversion in AVL and I

b) What is the diagnosis? *(1 mark)*
- Atrial fibrillation with pre-excitation (the key ECG finding to make the diagnosis of pre-excitation is the broad QRS of variable duration)

c) What ECG features suggest that a broad complex tachycardia is ventricular in origin? *(5 marks)*

  (1 mark for each correct feature to a maximum of 5)
- Atrioventricular (AV) dissociation
- QRS concordance throughout the chest leads
- Fusion beats
- Capture beats
- QRS >160 ms
- Extreme axis deviation
- Brugada sign
- Josephson sign

d) What is the definition of pre-excitation? *(2 marks)*
- The presence of an accessory pathway connecting the atria and ventricles ...
- ... allowing premature activation of the ventricle

e) Describe the potential resting ECG findings seen in a patient with an accessory pathway *(2 marks)*
- Sinus rhythm with a short PR interval and a delta wave, resulting in QRS >120 ms (typically representing an accessory pathway capable of antero- and retrograde conduction)
- Sinus rhythm with a normal PR interval and QRS morphology (a concealed pre-excitation pathway, typically only capable of retrograde conduction)

f) What pharmacological agents are used for the treatment of atrial fibrillation with pre-excitation in the haemodynamically stable patient? *(2 marks)*

(1 mark per agent to a maximum of 2)
- Procainamide
- Ibutilide
- Flecainide
- Propafenone

  (AV node-blocking antiarrhythmic drugs such as beta blockers, amiodarone, digoxin, adenosine, and verapamil should be avoided.)

g) What is the treatment for atrial fibrillation with pre-excitation in the haemodynamically unstable patient? *(1 mark)*
- Synchronized direct current (DC) cardioversion

h) Define the Wolff–Parkinson–White syndrome *(1 mark)*
- ECG evidence of an accessory pathway *and* symptomatic tachyarrhythmias

Notes

This is an example of a question where it would be easy to become disheartened if you had struggled with the 'ECG diagnosis'. This only contributes 1 mark out of a possible 20, and without it all subsequent marks are still available. Remember that the questions you remember aren't necessarily where the marks are to be found!

Further reading

Page RL, Joglar JA, Caldwell MA, Conti JB, Field ME, Hammill SC, et al. 2015 American College of Cardiology, American Heart Association and the Heart Rhythm Society guideline for the management of adult patients with supraventricular tachycardia. *Journal of the American College of Cardiology* 2016;67:1575–1623.

FFICM syllabus references 1.1, 2.3, 3.3, 4.1, 5.11.
CoBaTrICE domains 2, 3.

OSCE 8 station 5—data

Questions

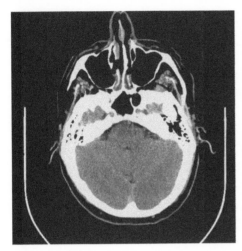 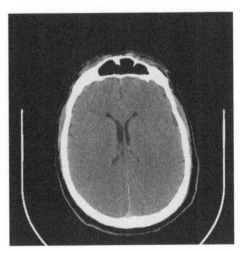

Figure 8.5 CT head

Reproduced from *The Comatose Patient, Second Edition*, Wijdicks EFM, Figure 65.1, Oxford University Press © 2014 Mayo Foundation for Medical Education and Research. Reproduced with permission of the Licensor through PLSclear

A 76-year-old man was admitted following an out-of-hospital cardiac arrest. He was intubated by paramedics at the scene after a long period without cardiopulmonary resuscitation. Coronary angiography revealed an occluded left main stem which was stented. He was managed with therapeutic hypothermia for 24 hours, after which sedation was stopped.

After 4 days on the critical care unit he was still not making any respiratory effort, had unreactive pupils and was not responding to painful stimuli. A computed tomography (CT) scan of his head was performed and is shown in Figure 8.5.

a) What are the significant abnormalities on the CT scan, and what is the most likely cause?
(*2 marks*)

After discussion with his family in the presence of the specialist nurse for organ donation, it is decided to perform brainstem death tests.

b) Who can perform brainstem death testing? (*2 marks*)
c) What preconditions must be met for brainstem death testing to take place? (*3 marks*)

d) Complete Table 8.1q to describe the cranial nerves (CNs) being examined during brainstem testing *(6 marks)*

Table 8.1q Brainstem tests and cranial nerves

Test	Sensory (afferent) CN	Motor (efferent) CN
Pupillary response		
Corneal reflexes		
Oculovestibular reflexes		
Response to painful stimulus		
Gag reflex		
Cough reflex		

e) Describe how the apnoea test is performed *(2 marks)*
f) What are the endocrine effects of losing brainstem function? *(3 marks)*
g) What additional requirements are there concerning who can perform brainstem tests in a child (>2 months of age)? *(2 marks)*

Answers

a) What are the significant abnormalities on the CT scan, and what is the most likely cause?
    (2 marks)
    • Diffuse cerebral oedema causing effacement of the basal cisterns and sulci. Loss of grey–white matter differentiation
    • Hypoxic brain injury

b) Who can perform brainstem death tests? *(2 marks)*
    • Qualified doctors who have been fully registered for at least 5 years, and are competent in the conduct and interpretation of brainstem death testing
    • One should be a consultant

c) What preconditions must be met for brainstem death testing to take place? *(3 marks)*
    • The patient should be deeply unconscious, apnoeic, and mechanically ventilated
    • There should be no doubt that the patient has suffered irreversible brain damage of known aetiology
    • The patient's condition must not, either completely or in part, be due to reversible influences such as sedative drugs, endocrine and metabolic abnormalities, hypothermia, or cardiovascular instability

d) Complete Table 8.1a to describe the cranial nerves (CNs) being examined during brainstem testing *(6 marks)*

Table 8.1a Brainstem tests and cranial nerves

Test	Sensory (afferent) CN	Motor (efferent) CN
Pupillary response	II	III
Corneal reflexes	V	VII
Oculovestibular reflexes	VIII	III, IV, VI
Response to painful stimulus	V	VII
Gag reflex	IX	X
Cough reflex	X	X

(1 mark for two correct answers to a maximum of 6)

e) Describe how the apnoea test is performed *(2 marks)*
    • The patient is pre-oxygenated and minute ventilation reduced to give a starting $PaCO_2$ ≥6.0 kPa and pH <7.4. The patient is then disconnected from the ventilator (oxygen can be insufflated to prevent hypoxaemia)
    • The patient is observed for at least 5 minutes for any signs of respiratory effort. At the end of the test, another arterial blood gas test is performed which must demonstrate an increase in the $PaCO_2$ of >0.5 kPa from the starting value

f) What are the endocrine effects of losing brainstem function? *(3 marks)*
    • Diabetes insipidus results from reduced levels of antidiuretic hormone following failure of the posterior pituitary
    • Reduced levels of triiodothyronine secondary to anterior pituitary failure
    • Reduced levels of cortisol due to failure of the anterior pituitary impairs the stress response. The consequent reduction of insulin secretion contributes to the development of hyperglycaemia

g) What additional requirements are there concerning who can perform brainstem tests in a child (>2 months of age)? *(2 marks)*

- One doctor should be a paediatrician
- One doctor should not be directly involved in the care of that patient

Further reading

Gardiner D, Manara A. Form for the diagnosis of death using neurological criteria (full guidance version). Available at: https://www.ficm.ac.uk/standards-and-guidelines/access-standards-and-guidelines [accessed 13 June 2018].

NHS Blood and Transplant. Diagnosing death using neurological criteria. An educational tool for healthcare professionals. Available at: https://www.odt.nhs.uk/deceased-donation/best-practice-guidance/donation-after-brainstem-death/diagnosing-death-using-neurological-criteria/ [accessed 13 June 2018].

Oram J, Murphy P. Diagnosis of death. *Continuing Education in Anaesthesia Critical Care & Pain* 2011;11:77–81.

FFICM syllabus references 2.1, 2.6, 3.6, 8.4, 8.5.
CoBaTrICE domains 2, 8.

OSCE 8 station 6—data

Questions

A researcher wants to know whether a drug improves survival. They decide to conduct a double-blinded randomized controlled trial.

a) What is a randomized controlled trial? *(3 marks)*
b) What is the difference between single, double, and triple blinding? *(3 marks)*
c) What is the null hypothesis for this study? *(1 mark)*
d) What is the difference between 'primary' and 'secondary' outcomes of a trial? *(2 marks)*

They define a level for statistical significance as $p < 0.05$.

e) What is a 'p-value'? *(1 mark)*

They calculate the chance of a false negative as 20% or 1:5.

f) What are the meanings of the terms 'false negative' and 'false positive'? *(2 marks)*
g) What is meant by the term 'study power' and what factors determine its value? *(2 marks)*
h) What is the power of this study, expressed as a percentage? *(1 mark)*

The results show a mortality rate of 20% in patients treated with the drug, and 30% in the control group. The p-value is 0.02.

i) What is the absolute risk reduction (ARR) for death? *(1 mark)*
j) What is the relative risk reduction (RRR) for death? *(1 mark)*
k) What is the meaning of the term 'number needed to treat' (NNT), and what is the NNT for this study? *(3 marks)*

Answers

a) What is a randomized controlled trial? *(3 marks)*
  - A research method in which similar people are randomly assigned to two (or more) groups
  - One group has the intervention being tested, the other has an alternative intervention, a dummy intervention (placebo), or no intervention at all
  - The groups are then compared, looking for new differences between them. This comparison is used to determine how effective the experimental intervention was

b) What is the difference between single, double, and triple blinding? *(3 marks)*

Blinding is keeping secret which group (intervention or control) an individual is allocated to.
  - Single blinding—only the subjects are blinded
  - Double blinding—the clinician/researcher is also blinded
  - Triple blinding—the individual or group analysing the data are also blinded

c) What is the null hypothesis for this study? *(1 mark)*
  - That there will be no difference (in this case in survival) between the groups

d) What is the difference between 'primary' and 'secondary' outcomes of a trial? *(2 marks)*
  - The primary outcome is the difference or change that the trial is designed to look for, in this example survival
  - Other differences between the groups might be found. These are secondary outcomes

e) What is a 'p-value'? *(1 mark)*
  - The p-value is the probability of observing results as extreme, or more extreme, than those observed if the null hypothesis is true

f) What are the meanings of the terms 'false negative' and 'false positive'? *(2 marks)*
  - Also called a type 2 or beta error, a false negative is incorrectly accepting the null hypothesis when there is a difference between the two groups
  - The opposite is a false positive (type 1 or alpha error), which is incorrectly rejecting the null hypothesis when there is no difference between the two groups

g) What is meant by the term 'study power' and what factors determine its value? *(2 marks)*
  - The power of a study is a measure of its ability to find a statistically significant difference
  - It depends on the actual difference between the groups (which usually must be estimated), the level at which a difference is considered 'significant' (the p-value) and the number of subjects in the study

h) What is the power of this study, expressed as a percentage? *(1 mark)*
  - Expressed as a percentage, the type 2 error is 100-power, therefore the power of this study is 80%

i) What is the absolute risk reduction (ARR) for death? *(1 mark)*
  - 10% (difference between the event rate in the two groups)

j) What is the relative risk reduction (RRR) for death? *(1 mark)*
  - 33% (ARR/control event rate)

k) What is the meaning of the term 'number needed to treat' (NNT), and what is the NNT for this study? *(3 marks)*
  - It is the number of subjects that would need to be subject to the intervention (on average) for one person to benefit
  - NNT is calculated as 100/ARR(%). In this example it is therefore 100/10 = 10

Notes

'Statistics questions' are often not looked forward to! The examiners are not asking you to be expert, but you would be expected to understand the key concepts that allow you to critically appraise a paper. If this is an area of weakness, dedicating some study time to this topic will be high yield both for your confidence and performance.

Further reading

Harris M, Taylor G. *Medical Statistics Made Easy*, 3rd Edition. Banbury: Scion Publishing; 2014.

FFICM syllabus references 11.6, 12.13, 12.15.
CoBaTrICE domains 11, 12.

OSCE 8 station 7—data

Questions

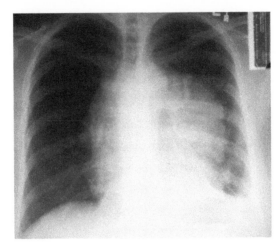

Figure 8.6 Chest X-ray

Reproduced from Lipschik, G., Feldt, J., et al., *Oxford American Handbook of Clinical Diagnosis* (2009), with permission from Oxford University Press

A patient is admitted to hospital for investigation of weight loss and dyspnoea. Their chest X-ray is shown in Figure 8.6.

a) What is the most striking abnormality on the chest X-ray? *(1 mark)*

b) What are the common causes of unilateral hilar opacification? *(3 marks)*

A mediastinal lymph node biopsy confirms lymphoma. The patient is started on chemotherapy and a week later develops oral paraesthesia, muscle cramps, and spasms. Blood tests reveal hyperkalaemia and hypocalcaemia.

c) What other neurological signs might be seen in a patient with acute hypocalcaemia? *(3 marks)*

d) What is the most likely diagnosis? *(1 mark)*

e) What are some common risk factors for the development of tumour lysis syndrome (TLS)? *(3 marks)*

f) Which other plasma biochemical parameters may be elevated in TLS? *(3 marks)*

g) What treatment should be given for TLS? *(5 marks)*

h) What is the role of allopurinol in the management of TLS? *(1 mark)*

Answers

a) What is the most striking abnormality on the chest X-ray? *(1 mark)*
   - Left hilar opacification

b) What are the common causes of unilateral hilar opacification? *(3 marks)*

   (1 mark per cause to a maximum of 3)
   - Solid organ tumours—bronchial carcinoma or metastases
   - Haematological malignancy—lymphoma
   - Infection—primary TB, fungal infection, atypical mycobacteria, viral
   - Sarcoidosis

c) What other neurological signs might be seen in a patient with acute hypocalcaemia? *(3 marks)*

   (1 mark per cause to a maximum of 3)
   - Acral paraesthesia
   - Trousseau's sign
   - Chvostek's sign
   - Hyperreflexia
   - Generalized tetany
   - Seizures
   - Papilloedema
   - Acute psychiatric disturbance

d) What is the most likely diagnosis? *(1 mark)*
   - Tumour lysis syndrome

e) What are some common risk factors for the development of tumour lysis syndrome (TLS)? *(3 marks)*

   (1 mark per cause to a maximum of 3)
   - Increased age
   - Pre-existing renal impairment or renal involvement by tumour
   - Dehydration
   - High tumour burden
   - High-grade tumours with rapid cell turnover
   - Highly chemosensitive tumour
   - Use of medication that increase uric acid levels

f) Which other plasma biochemical parameters may be elevated in TLS? *(3 marks)*

   (1 mark per cause to a maximum of 3)
   - Uric acid
   - Phosphate
   - Urea
   - Creatinine
   - Lactate dehydrogenase

g) What treatment should be given for TLS? *(5 marks)*
   - Vigorous hydration maintaining polyuria
   - Correction of symptomatic hypocalcaemia
   - Medical management of hyperkalaemia
   - Management of hyperuricaemia with drugs such as rasburicase
   - Renal replacement therapy if indicated (fluid overload, acute kidney injury, or electrolyte disturbances refractory to medical management)

h) What is the role of allopurinol in the management of TLS? *(1 mark)*
  - Allopurinol is a prophylactic agent used in the prevention of uric acid deposition but does not affect breakdown of uric acid once TLS is established

Further reading

Jones GL, Will A, Jackson GH, Webb NJA, Rule S, British Committee for Standards in Haematology. Guidelines for the management of tumour lysis syndrome in adults and children with haematological malignancies on behalf of the British Committee for Standards in Haematology. *British Journal of Haematology* 2015;169:661–671.

FFICM syllabus references 2.1, 2.2, 2.6, 3.1, 3.2, 3.4, 4.1, 4.7, 4.8.
CoBaTrICE domains 1, 2, 3.

OSCE 8 station 8—data

Questions

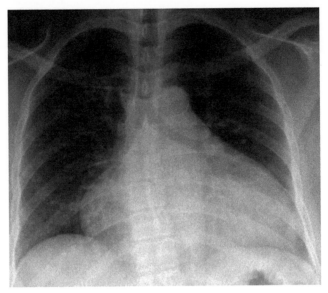

Figure 8.7 Chest X-ray

A 70-year-old man has been admitted to hospital with a 5-week history of fatigue and dyspnoea. On examination he has quiet heart sounds and an elevated jugular venous pressure.

Look at Figure 8.7.

a) What is the most significant abnormality on this chest X-ray? *(1 mark)*

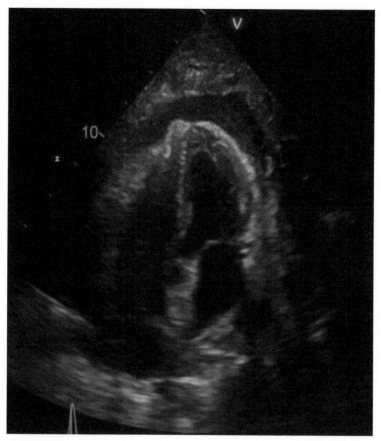

Figure 8.8 Echocardiogram

An echocardiogram is performed to investigate the enlarged cardiac shadow (Figure 8.8).

b) What abnormality is shown on this apical four-chamber image? *(1 mark)*

c) How can pericardial effusions be classified in terms of their size? *(3 marks)*

d) What are the potential causes of pericardial effusions? *(6 marks)*

The next day the patient complains of feeling faint and his respiratory rate increases to 34 breaths per minute. His observations show a sinus tachycardia and hypotension. You notice that his radial pulse weakens during inspiration.

e) What clinical scenario has developed? *(1 mark)*

f) Other than tachycardia, what electrocardiographic changes are commonly seen in cardiac tamponade? *(2 marks)*

g) What is pulsus paradoxus? *(2 marks)*

h) What options are available for the treatment of acute cardiac tamponade? *(2 marks)*

i) In which clinical scenarios would surgical drainage of pericardial tamponade be the preferred option? *(2 marks)*

Answers

a) What is the most significant abnormality on this chest X-ray? *(1 mark)*
  • Symmetrically enlarged cardiac silhouette

b) What abnormality is shown on this apical four-chamber image? *(1 mark)*
  • Pericardial effusion

c) How can pericardial effusions be classified in terms of their size? *(3 marks)*
  • Mild—<10 mm
  • Moderate—10–20 mm
  • Severe—>20 mm

d) What are the potential causes of pericardial effusions? *(6 marks)*

  (1 mark per cause to a maximum of 6)
  • Infective—bacterial, viral, fungal, or parasitic
  • Autoimmune—lupus, rheumatoid arthritis
  • Traumatic/iatrogenic
  • Inflammatory—post myocardial infarction or surgery
  • Neoplastic
  • Drug related
  • Metabolic—hypothyroidism, uraemia
  • Idiopathic

e) What clinical scenario has developed? *(1 mark)*
  • Cardiac tamponade

f) Other than tachycardia, what electrocardiographic changes are commonly seen in cardiac tamponade? *(2 marks)*
  • Small QRS complexes
  • Electrical alternans

g) What is pulsus paradoxus? *(2 marks)*
  • A decrease in systolic blood pressure during inspiration …
  • … of >10 mmHg

h) What options are available for the treatment of acute cardiac tamponade? *(2 marks)*
  • Needle pericardiocentesis
  • Surgical drainage

i) In which clinical scenarios would surgical drainage of pericardial tamponade be the preferred option? *(2 marks)*

  (1 mark per scenario to a maximum of 2)
  • Intrapericardial bleeding
  • Clot within the pericardium
  • Loculated effusion

Further reading

Katritsis D, Gersh B, Camm AJ. Pericardial effusion and cardiac tamponade. In: *Clinical Cardiology Current Practice Guidelines*, 4th Edition, pp. 516–521. Oxford: Oxford University Press; 2016.

FFICM syllabus references 1.1, 2.6, 3.3, 5.13.
CoBaTrICE domains 1, 2, 4, 5.

OSCE 8 station 9—data

Questions

You are asked to review a 50-year-old obese woman with pancreatitis. Her blood pressure is 85/30 mmHg and she has only passed 50 mL of urine in the last 4 hours despite adequate fluid resuscitation. You notice that her serum creatinine has been double her baseline value for over 48 hours and that her serum amylase is 950 IU/dL (normal range: 0–180 IU/dL).

a) What feature of this clinical scenario defines the pancreatitis as being severe? *(1 mark)*
b) What is the significance of obesity in acute pancreatitis? *(2 marks)*
c) Why should an ultrasound examination be performed in cases of confirmed pancreatitis? *(2 marks)*

An abdominal ultrasound is performed which shows a dilated common bile duct with no visible stone. 'Sludge' is seen in the gallbladder.

d) What intervention should be performed? *(1 mark)*

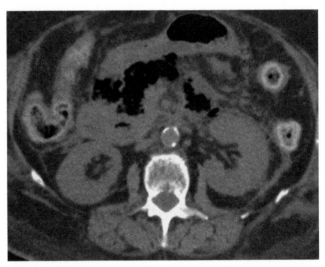

Figure 8.9 CT abdomen

During the 24 hours following endoscopic retrograde cholangiopancreatography (ERCP) the patient developed acute respiratory distress and required invasive ventilation. Because of this deterioration, a computed tomography (CT) scan of the abdomen was performed and is shown in Figure 8.9.

e) What features, if found on CT, are associated with an increased severity of pancreatitis? *(3 marks)*
f) What feature of this image suggests that the necrotic areas are infected? *(1 mark)*
g) Other than ensuring appropriate antibiotic treatment, what other interventions should be considered in the context of infected pancreatic necrosis? *(3 marks)*

h) Complete Table 8.2q to define the pancreatic and peripancreatic collections for each description *(4 marks)*

Table 8.2q Pancreatic and peripancreatic fluid collections

Usually resolve spontaneously Confined by normal tissue planes Homogeneous
Occurs >4 weeks after onset of symptoms Intrapancreatic and/or extrapancreatic Heterogeneous
Occurs >4 weeks after onset of symptoms Encapsulated Homogeneous
Absent wall Occurs in the presence of necrosis Heterogeneous

i) What surgical intervention will be required as soon as possible after this patient has recovered from her pancreatitis? *(1 mark)*
j) What long-term pancreatic complications are likely in this patient? *(2 marks)*

Answers

a) What feature of this clinical scenario defines the pancreatitis as being severe? *(1 mark)*
- Organ failure not resolving within 48 hours

b) What is the significance of obesity in acute pancreatitis? *(2 marks)*
- Pancreatitis is more prevalent in the obese
- Obesity is associated with an increased severity of disease

c) Why should an ultrasound examination be performed in cases of confirmed pancreatitis? *(2 marks)*
- To demonstrate the presence/absence of gallstones ...
- ... and/or common bile duct dilation

d) What intervention should be performed? *(1 mark)*
- Therapeutic endoscopic retrograde cholangiopancreatography

e) What features, if found on CT, are associated with an increased severity of pancreatitis? *(3 marks)*
- Extensive fat stranding
- Peri-pancreatitis fluid collections
- Necrosis of the pancreas

f) What feature of this image suggests that the necrotic areas are infected? *(1 mark)*
- The presence of gas in the pancreas and peri-pancreatic tissues

g) Other than ensuring appropriate antibiotic treatment, what other interventions should be considered in the context of infected pancreatic necrosis? *(3 marks)*
- Fine needle aspiration for culture
- Percutaneous drainage
- Surgical necrosectomy

h) Complete Table 8.2a to define the pancreatic and peripancreatic collections for each description *(4 marks)*

Table 8.2a Pancreatic and peripancreatic fluid collections

Usually resolve spontaneously Confined by normal tissue planes Homogeneous	*Acute peripancreatic fluid collection*
Occurs >4 weeks after onset of symptoms Intrapancreatic and/or extrapancreatic Heterogeneous	*Walled-off necrosis*
Occurs >4 weeks after onset of symptoms Encapsulated Homogeneous	*Pancreatic pseudocyst*
Absent wall Occurs in the presence of necrosis Heterogeneous	*Acute necrotic collection*

i) What surgical intervention will be required as soon as possible after this patient has recovered from her pancreatitis? *(1 mark)*
- Cholecystectomy

j) What long-term pancreatic complications are likely in this patient? *(2 marks)*
- Exocrine deficiency requiring pancreatic digestive enzyme supplementation
- Diabetes mellitus

Further reading

UK Working Party on Acute Pancreatitis. UK guidelines for the management of acute pancreatitis. *Gut* 2005;54(Suppl III):iii1–iii9.

Banks PA, Bollen TL, Dervenis C, Gooszen HG, Johnson CD, Sarr MG, et al. Classification of acute pancreatitis— 2012: revision of the Atlanta classification and definitions by international consensus. *Gut* 2013;62:102–111.

FFICM syllabus references 2.6, 3.1, 3.7, 6.1.
CoBaTrICE domains 2, 3, 4.

OSCE 8 station 10—data

Questions

a) With respect to arterial blood gases, what is the definition of base excess (BE)? *(3 marks)*

b) How does the standard base excess (SBE) differ from BE, and what is the rationale for this difference? *(2 marks)*

c) What is the unit of measurement for base excess? *(1 mark)*

A normally well patient presents with diabetic ketoacidosis. Her arterial bicarbonate concentration is measured as 10 mmol/L (24–30 mmol/L).

d) What is the primary acid–base disturbance? *(1 mark)*

e) Using the Boston rules for arterial blood gas interpretation, what would you expect her $PaCO_2$ to be? *(2 marks)*

The measured $PaCO_2$ is 3.0 (normal range: 4.7–6.0 kPa).

f) What is the clinical usefulness of calculating an expected $PaCO_2$ in metabolic acidosis? *(2 marks)*

g) What additional information is required to calculate this patient's anion gap? *(1 mark)*

The patient is resuscitated using 0.9% sodium chloride solution. Blood tests taken after this resuscitation show:

- Sodium 140 mmol/L (normal range: 135–145 mmol/L)
- Chloride 115 mmol/L (normal range: 95–105 mmol/L)

h) Using the Stewart approach, what is the sodium/chloride BE effect? *(2 marks)*

i) What term is used to describe to the finding of a negative sodium/chloride BE effect? *(1 mark)*

A second patient presents with acute respiratory distress. They have no known comorbidities. An arterial blood gas test reveals acidaemia and a $PaCO_2$ of 9.3 kPa (4.7–6.0 kPa).

j) Using the Boston rules, what would you expect this patient's bicarbonate concentration to be? *(4 marks)*

k) The patient has a measured bicarbonate concentration of 23 mmol/L. What does this lower than expected value suggest about the acid–base disturbance? *(1 mark)*

Answers

a) With respect to arterial blood gasses, what is the definition of base excess (BE)? *(3 marks)*
   - The amount of acid or base required to restore 1 L of blood to a pH of 7.4 ...
   - ... at a PCO_2 of 5.3 kPa ...
   - ... and at body temperature

b) How does the standard base excess (SBE) differ from BE, and what is the rationale for this difference? *(2 marks)*
   - The standard base deficit is corrected to a haemoglobin concentration of 50 g/dL and is defined in terms of a litre of extracellular fluid
   - This correction allows for a better reflection of the acid–base status of the whole body. Haemoglobin acts as a buffer in the blood but not in the interstitial space, so measuring a BE at the patient's haemoglobin concentration (assuming it is >50 g/dL) overestimates the degree of buffering *in vivo*

c) What is the unit of measurement for BE? *(1 mark)*
   - mEq/L

d) What is the primary acid–base disturbance? *(1 mark)*
   - Acidaemia

e) Using the Boston rules for arterial blood gas interpretation, what would you expect her $PaCO_2$ to be? *(2 marks)*
   - In a metabolic acidosis, expected $PaCO_2$ (kPa) = 0.2[bicarbonate] +1 (+/− 0.3)
   - $PaCO_2$ = 2.7–3.3 kPa

f) What is the clinical usefulness of calculating an expected $PaCO_2$ in metabolic acidosis? *(2 marks)*
   - Assesses for a coexisting respiratory alkalosis or acidosis
   - May help in deciding ventilator settings once physiological adaptation has been taken away

g) What additional information is required to calculate this patient's anion gap? *(1 mark)*
   - Serum concentrations of sodium, potassium, and chloride

h) Using the Stewart approach, what is the sodium/chloride BE effect? *(2 marks)*
   - Na/Cl BE effect = (measured [Na] − measured [Cl]) − 40
   - Na/Cl BE effect = (140 − 115) − 40 = −15

i) What term is used to describe to the finding of a negative sodium/chloride base excess effect? *(1 mark)*
   - Hyperchloraemic acidosis

j) Using the Boston rules, what would you expect this patient's bicarbonate concentration to be? *(4 marks)*
   - In respiratory acidosis, a 1 kPa increase in $PaCO_2$ causes a 0.75 mmol/L increase in bicarbonate concentration
   - 0.75 × (9.3 − 5.3) = 3
   - Normal bicarbonate concentration = 24–30 mmol/L
   - Expected bicarbonate concentration = 27–33 mmol/L

k) The patient has a measured bicarbonate concentration of 23 mmol/L. What does this lower than expected value suggest about the acid–base disturbance? *(1 mark)*

   - There is a coexisting metabolic acidosis

Notes

This question is a bit of a stinker. Practising it demonstrates several things, however.

1. You might be thrown a curveball in the exam, one of the skills of the OSCE is the ability to forget about it and move on, but also to not give up on a question and achieve the easier marks hidden within the question
2. For very familiar topics (such as arterial blood gases), it's worth expanding your knowledge but also making sure you really do know the basics (e.g. definition of BE)

Further reading

Story D. Stewart acid-base: a simplified bedside approach. *Anesthesia & Analgesia* 2016;123:511–515.

FFICM syllabus references 2.2, 2.5, 2.8.
CoBaTrICE domains 2.

OSCE 8 station 11—data

Questions

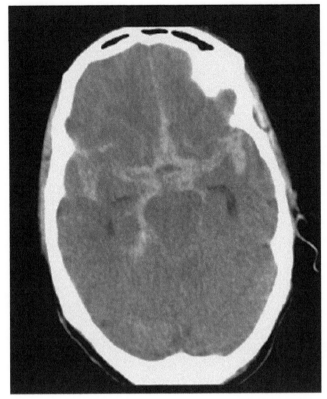

Figure 8.10 CT head

Reproduced from *Oxford Textbook of Neurocritical Care*, Smith M *et al.*, Fig 18.1. © 2016 Oxford University Press. Reproduced with permission of the Licensor through PLSclear

Look at the computed tomography (CT) image in Figure 8.10.

a) What abnormal findings are shown on this image? *(2 marks)*

b) What is the commonest cause of a spontaneous subarachnoid haemorrhage? *(1 mark)*

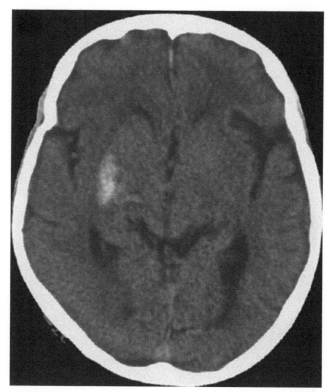

Figure 8.11 CT head

Reproduced from *Oxford Textbook of Neurocritical Care*, Smith M *et al.*, Fig 19.1. © 2016 Oxford University Press. Reproduced with permission of the Licensor through PLSclear

Look at Figure 8.11.

c) What abnormal findings are shown on this image? *(1 mark)*

d) What is the most common cause of an intracerebral haemorrhage? *(1 mark)*

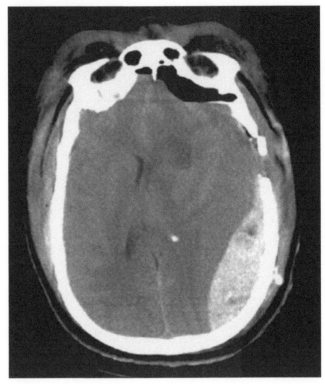

Figure 8.12 CT head

Look at Figure 8.12.

e) What abnormal findings are shown on this image? *(4 marks)*

f) What is the commonest mechanism for extradural haemorrhage? *(1 mark)*

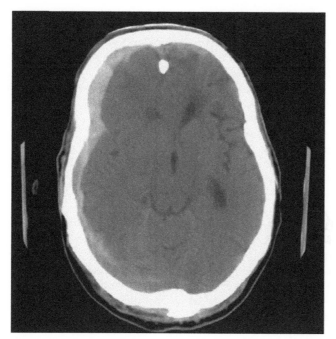

Figure 8.13 CT head

Reproduced from *Oxford Textbook of Neurocritical Care*, Smith M *et al.*, Fig 17.1. © 2016 Oxford University Press. Reproduced with permission of the Licensor through PLSclear

Look at Figure 8.13.

g) How would you describe the abnormalities on this image? *(2 marks)*

h) What is the commonest vascular cause of a subdural haemorrhage? *(1 mark)*

i) According to Brain Trauma Foundation guidelines, what should be the target systolic blood pressure and cerebral perfusion pressure after traumatic brain injury? *(3 marks)*

j) According to the Brain Trauma Foundation, what are the four non-radiological early predictors of poor prognosis in traumatic brain injury? *(4 marks)*

Answers

a) What abnormal findings are shown on this image? *(2 marks)*
- Subarachnoid haemorrhage ...
- ... with blood in the suprasellar and ambient cisterns

b) What is the commonest cause of a spontaneous subarachnoid haemorrhage? *(1 mark)*
- Rupture of an intracranial saccular aneurysm

c) What abnormal findings are shown on this image? *(1 mark)*
- Right-sided intracerebral haemorrhage

d) What is the most common cause of an intracerebral haemorrhage? *(1 mark)*
- Spontaneous rupture of small intracerebral arteries or arterioles, most commonly due to hypertension

e) What abnormal findings are shown on this image? *(4 marks)*
- Large left-sided occipitoparietal extradural haematoma
- Fractured skull in the temporoparietal region
- Midline shift with subfalcine herniation
- Pneumocranium

f) What is the commonest cause of extradural haemorrhage? *(1 mark)*
- Traumatic arterial bleed between the dura mater and cranium

g) How would you describe the abnormalities on this image? *(2 marks)*
- Right-sided acute subdural haematoma
- Midline shift with ipsilateral loss of the Sylvian fissure and sulci

h) What is the commonest vascular cause of a subdural haemorrhage? *(1 mark)*
- Tearing of a bridging vein between the cerebral cortex and a draining venous sinus leading to bleeding between the dura and arachnoid mater

i) According to Brain Trauma Foundation guidelines, what should be the target systolic blood pressure (SBP) and cerebral perfusion pressure after traumatic brain injury? *(3 marks)*
- SBP ≥100 mmHg for patients aged 50–69 years
- SBP ≥110 mmHg for patients aged 5–49 or >69 years
- Cerebral perfusion pressure between 60 and 70 mmHg

j) According to the Brain Trauma Foundation, what are the four non-radiological early predictors of poor prognosis in traumatic brain injury? *(4 marks)*
- Glasgow Coma Score
- Age
- Bilaterally absent pupillary light reflex
- Hypotension (SBP <90 mmHg)

Further reading

Brain Trauma Foundation. Guidelines for the management of severe traumatic brain injury, fourth edition. Available at: https://braintrauma.org/uploads/07/04/Guidelines_for_the_Management_of_Severe_Traumatic.97250_ _2_.pdf [accessed 7 February 2018].

FFICM syllabus references 1.5, 2.6, 2.7, 3.1, 3.6, 11.6.
CoBaTrICE domains 2, 3.

OSCE 8 station 12—equipment

Questions

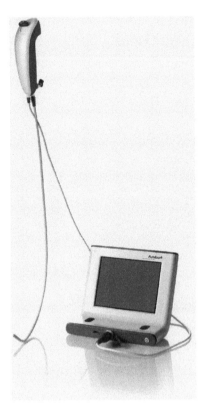

Figure 8.14 Medical device
Image courtesy of Ambu USA, Glen Burnie, MD

Look at Figure 8.14.

a) What is this piece of equipment? *(1 mark)*

b) How is an image generated by a single-use bronchoscope? *(1 mark)*

c) What are the potential advantages of single-use bronchoscopes on the intensive care unit?
(4 marks)

d) After use, what processes should a reusable fibreoptic bronchoscope undergo prior to reuse?
(6 marks)

e) What pathogen is most commonly reported in cases of bronchoscopic contamination despite good cleaning practice? *(1 mark)*

f) What is the difference between cleaning, disinfection, and sterilization? *(3 marks)*

g) What methods are available for sterilizing medical equipment? *(4 marks)*

Answers

a) What is this piece of equipment? (*1 mark*)
   - Single-use flexible bronchoscope

b) How is an image generated by a single-use bronchoscope? (*1 mark*)
   - A distal camera illuminated by a light-emitting diode

c) What are the potential advantages of single-use bronchoscopes in the intensive care unit?
   (*4 marks*)

   (1 mark per advantage to a maximum of 4)
   - No risk of cross-contamination from other patients
   - Immediately available
   - Reduced upfront capital costs
   - No maintenance costs from servicing or cleaning
   - Less potential for damage as no transit for cleaning and processing
   - Less staff workload in arranging reuse process

d) After use, what processes should a reusable fibreoptic bronchoscope undergo prior to reuse?
   (*6 marks*)
   - Clean debris and flush all lumens
   - Disassembly and inspection for defects
   - Leak test
   - Manual or automated chemical sterilization
   - Rinsing and drying
   - Upright storage in a disassembled form

e) What pathogen is most commonly reported in cases of bronchoscopic contamination despite good cleaning practice? (*1 mark*)
   - *Mycobacterium tuberculosis*

f) What is the difference between cleaning, disinfection, and sterilization? (*3 marks*)
   - Cleaning is the removal of visible contamination
   - Disinfection is the removal of organisms that have potential to cause infection, excluding spores and some viruses
   - Sterilization is the removal of all microbials including spores

g) What methods are available for sterilizing medical equipment? (*4 marks*)

   - Dry heat, e.g. hot air oven, baking, incineration
   - Moist heat sterilization, e.g. autoclave
   - Chemical sterilization, e.g. ethylene oxide
   - Irradiation, e.g. ultraviolet

Further reading

Yoo JH. Review of disinfection and sterilization—back to the basics. *Infection and Chemotherapy* 2018;50:101–109.

FFICM syllabus references 5.5, 11.2, 11.3.
CoBaTrICE domains 5, 11.

OSCE 8 station 13—equipment

Questions

A patient on the intensive care unit has suffered a micro-shock resulting in ventricular fibrillation (VF).

a) What must be present for a micro-shock to occur? *(2 marks)*

A defibrillator is used to deliver a biphasic shock with an energy of 150 J.

b) What is the advantage of a biphasic waveform? *(1 mark)*
c) What is the relationship between the delivered current and thoracic impedance? *(1 mark)*

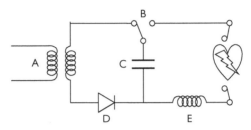

Figure 8.15 Defibrillator circuit

Look at Figure 8.15.

d) Complete Table 8.3q to identify the components of the defibrillator circuit and to describe their purpose *(10 marks)*

Table 8.3q Components of a defibrillator circuit

Component	Purpose
A	
B	
C	
D	
E	

e) What medications and strategies can be considered to treat refractory VF? *(5 marks)*
f) How far should a defibrillator pad be placed from a permanent pacemaker? *(1 mark)*

Answers

a) What must be present for a micro-shock to occur? *(2 marks)*
   - A direct pathway for an electrical current to reach the myocardium
   - A current source

b) What is the advantage of a biphasic waveform? *(1 mark)*
   - A biphasic waveform enables more effective defibrillation at a lower energy (lower defibrillation threshold) when compared with monophasic waveforms

c) What is the relationship between the delivered current and thoracic impedance? *(1 mark)*
   - Delivered current = 1/thoracic impedance

d) Complete Table 8.3a to identify the components of the defibrillator circuit and to describe their purpose *(10 marks)*

Table 8.3a Components of a defibrillator circuit

	Component	Purpose
A	Transformer	Increases the potential difference
B	Switch	Determines whether the energy can enter the patient circuit
C	Capacitor	Stores the electrical energy
D	Rectifier/diode	Converts the current from alternating to direct current
E	Inductor coil	Delays and modifies the discharge

e) What medications and strategies can be considered to treat refractory VF? *(5 marks)*

   (1 mark per medication/strategy to a maximum of 4)
   - Amiodarone
   - Lidocaine
   - Magnesium
   - Esmolol
   - Movement of pads
   - Stacked shocks
   - Increased defibrillation energy
   - Double sequential defibrillation
   - Radiofrequency ablation
   - Extracorporeal membrane oxygenation

f) How far should a defibrillator pad be placed from a permanent pacemaker? *(1 mark)*
   - At least 8 cm

Notes

While you won't be expected to produce a wiring diagram for every piece of equipment you use, the defibrillator circuit is a clinically orientated way of testing some basic physics.

Further reading

Jacobs I, Sunde K, Deakin CD, Hazinski MF, Kerber RE, Koster RW, et al. 2010 International consensus on cardiopulmonary resuscitation and emergency cardiovascular care science with treatment recommendations Part 6: Defibrillation. *Circulation* 2010;122(Suppl 2): S325–S337.

FFICM syllabus references 1.2, 5.11, 11.3.
CoBaTrICE domains 1, 5.

Index